Metabolic and Nutritional Disorders in the Elderly

Edited by
A. N. Exton-Smith MA MD FRCP
Barlow Professor of Geriatric Medicine, University College Hospital Medical School; Honorary Consultant Physician, University College Hospital, London

and
F. I. Caird MA DM FRCP
David Cargill Professor of Geriatric Medicine, University of Glasgow

With a Foreword by
Sir Ferguson Anderson OBE MD FRCP FRFPS KStJ
Formerly Professor of Geriatric Medicine, University of Glasgow

A JOHN WRIGHT & SONS LTD PUBLICATION
Distributed by
YEAR BOOK MEDICAL PUBLISHERS, INC.
35 E. Wacker Drive · Chicago

Published by John Wright & Sons Ltd, 42–44 Triangle West, Bristol BS8 1EX

Distributed in the United States of America by
YEAR BOOK MEDICAL PUBLISHERS, INC.

(ISBN: 0–8151–1405–2)

by arrangement with
JOHN WRIGHT & SONS LTD.

Printed in Great Britain by Billing & Sons Ltd,
Guildford, London and Worcester.

Preface

The increasing numbers of old people in developed Western societies, and the increasing levels of disability that they show with advancing age, present increasing problems to the medical and social agencies upon which they rely for help. The metabolic and endocrine disorders of old age are of especial importance in this context, because, by contrast with essentially structural conditions, such as for instance cerebral or cardiac infarction, they are usually eminently amenable to treatment, and capable of true improvement, if properly diagnosed and assessed. There remain many difficulties of interpretation in the nutrition of the elderly, despite much excellent work in recent years, while understanding of the common endocrine disorders, such as diabetes and thyroid disease, has outstripped knowledge of the basic processes of ageing in the organs concerned. In the present volume we have tried to set out both the fundamental scientific aspects of these disorders as they are at present understood, and the practical diagnostic and therapeutic considerations, as they are seen by experts in the fields in question. We hope that the results of this approach will be of value both to physicians interested in the care of the elderly, and to those concerned with the general problems of ageing in man.

A.N.E-S.
F.I.C.

Contributors

G. A. Bray MD
Professor of Medicine, UCLA School of Medicine,
Harbor-UCLA Medical Center, Torrance, California, USA

F. I. Caird MA DM FRCP
David Cargill Professor of Geriatric Medicine,
University of Glasgow

Molly M. Disselduff, BSc (Syd) Dip Diet
Principal Research Officer (Nutrition),
Department of Health and Social Security, London

A. N. Exton-Smith MA MD FRCP
Barlow Professor of Geriatric Medicine,
University College Hospital Medical School, London

J. H. Fuller MA MRCP
Senior Research Fellow, Department of Medical Statistics and Epidemiology,
London School of Hygiene and Tropical Medicine

M. H. N. Golden BSc MB MRCP
Wellcome Trust Senior Research Fellow; Senior Lecturer, Department of Nutrition,
London School of Hygiene and Tropical Medicine

M. F. Green MA MB BChir MRCP
Consultant Physician, Department of Geriatric Medicine,
Royal Free Hospital, London

D. Heber MD PhD
Assistant Professor of Medicine, UCLA School of Medicine,
Harbor-UCLA Medical Center, Torrance, California, USA

M. Hodkinson MA DM FRCP
Professor of Geriatric Medicine,
Royal Postgraduate Medical School, London

D. E. Hyams MB FRCP
Medical Director, Clinical Research International,
Merck, Sharp & Dohme Research Laboratories, Rahway, New Jersey, USA

T. G. Judge MB ChB FRCP
Consultant Physician in Geriatric Medicine,
Royal Infirmary and Longmore Hospital, Edinburgh

H. Keen MD FRCP
Professor of Human Metabolism, and Director, Unit for Metabolic Medicine,
Guy's Hospital, London

H. N. Munro MB DSc
Scientific Director, USDA Human Nutrition Center,
Tufts University, Boston, USA

B. E. C. Nordin MD FRCP DSc
Professor of Mineral Metabolism,
University of Leeds

J. Runcie MB ChB FRCP
Consultant Physician,
University Department of Geriatric Medicine, Glasgow

J. A. Thomson MD PhD FRCP
Consultant Endocrinologist,
Glasgow Royal Infirmary

S. G. P. Webster MA MD MRCP
Consultant Physician in General and Geriatric Medicine,
Cambridge District Hospitals

V. R. Young PhD
Professor of Nutritional Biochemistry,
Massachusetts Institute of Technology, Cambridge, Massachusetts, USA

Contents

Foreword

The rapid progress made over the last decade in the understanding of metabolic disorders in the elderly justifies the publication of this important book. It is also true that the appreciation of our previous lack of information regarding the nutritional intake and requirements of older people imply that the time is ripe for a review of the present state of knowledge. From the earliest recorded history of medicine it was realized that bones become thin in old age but only relatively recently have modern methods of investigation been applied to this vital problem. The wide range of topics covered in this international text demonstrate its potential value and this is fully appreciated when the views of the experts are read. I feel greatly honoured by being invited to write these few words of introduction and am completely convinced of the relevance and importance of the subjects discussed. This work demonstrates the continuing need for the scientific approach to the many aspects of this fascinating subject of Geriatric Medicine.

Sir Ferguson Anderson

1. ENERGY REQUIREMENTS
D. Heber and G. A. Bray

Man as he ages undergoes a host of structural and functional changes considered part of the normal course of human development. In addition, elderly individuals have an increased incidence of heart disease, diabetes mellitus, cancer, osteoporosis, and other entities labelled as chronic or degenerative diseases (Eckstein, 1973; Anderson, 1974). Such illnesses are not always susceptible to the acute remedies of modern medicine, and increasing attention has been directed at preventive approaches to these diseases, of which correction of nutritional deficiencies among the elderly is of prime importance. Nutritional deficiencies have been implicated in the aetiology of many diseases of the aged (Dreizen, 1974), and nutritional deficiencies in the elderly population as a whole have been well-documented (Kaplan et al., 1955; Chope and Breslow, 1956; Steinkamp et al., 1965). This chapter will examine energy requirements and homeostasis in the aged and attempt to develop some desirable nutritional goals for the elderly based on observed changes with ageing in nutrition, body composition, and energy-requiring processes.

ENERGY HOMEOSTASIS
The process of energy homeostasis maintains a dynamic balance between nutrient intake and energy expenditure. This highly complex process begins with the interaction of the organism with its environment resulting from the intake of nutrients. These nutrients flow into various body compartments and into cells of those compartments under the control of neural and hormonal stimuli. These stimuli are to some extent dependent on the level of nutrient intake and during periods of low intake act to mobilize energy stored within body compartments as carbohydrate, fat and protein. Such fuels, whether from exogenous nutrients or endogenous energy stores, are metabolized to produce the energy for mechanical work and for the processes measured as the basal metabolic rate (BMR). The latter processes include the maintenance of a constant internal temperature; the maintenance of the intracellular environment via ion-pumping and protein synthesis; and the mechanical processes such as respiration and cardiac function which sustain the body at rest. Operationally, the BMR is measured 12–18 hours after a meal in a neutral thermal environment by direct or indirect measurement of oxygen consumption (Consolazio et al., 1963).

1

As shown in *Fig.* 1.1, adenosine triphospahte (ATP) is the principal chemical intermediate for energy transfer in the body. The energy of ATP contained within the high energy bond of the terminal phosphate can be coupled to biochemical or physical processes with the subsequent formation of adenosine diphosphate (ADP). ATP supplies can be regenerated from ADP via the process of oxidative phosphorylation. The details of oxidative phosphorylation are outside the scope of this chapter, but the net result is that water and carbon dioxide are produced while oxygen and fuels are

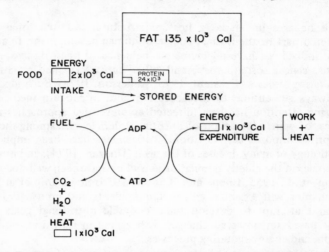

Fig. 1.1 Fuel storage and utilization. The relationship between the intake of energy, the size of the storage depots, and the overall pathway for the generation of ATP is depicted. Only about half of the energy that is ingested is actually stored as the high energy intermediary ATP, the rest being dissipated as heat.

consumed in the process of ATP formation. The process of fuel combustion results in half the total fuel energy being released as heat and half the energy being captured in the terminal phosphate bond of ATP. The transfer of energy from ATP to biochemical and physical processes also results in the liberation of heat. Heat from both the formation and degradation of ATP plays a role in the maintenance of internal temperature.

In man, the principal endogenous fuel reservoir is fat, which contains approximately 135 000 kcal*. Protein stores, primarily in muscle, represent 24 000 kcal, while liver glycogen and other carbohydrate stores represent only 1200 kcal (Moore and Brennan, 1974). All of these fuels can be utilized to regenerate ATP stores when nutrient intake is lowered (*Fig.* 1.2). Triglycerides from the diet or fat stores ultimately yield fatty acids and glycerol. Glycerol may be returned to the liver to form glucose, and under certain circumstances, fatty acids can be converted to ketones by the liver.

*1 kcal = 4·2 kJ.

Dietary polysaccharides and stored glycogen can be converted to glucose. Finally, protein from the diet or body cells can be broken down to amino acids. These circulating metabolites enter the liver mitochondria where, via the Krebs cycle, oxidative phosphorylation is promoted with the formation of ATP, carbon dioxide, water and heat. Fatty acids and ketones are converted to acetyl coenzyme A in the liver. Glucose, lactate and some amino acids are converted to pyruvate and then to acetyl coenzyme A. Other amino acids enter the Krebs cycle directly and the ammonia released

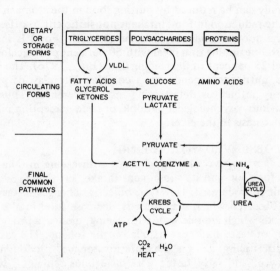

Fig. 1.2. Food sources and the overview of metabolism. Fats, proteins and carbohydrates are the macronutrients of the diet. When they are digested and absorbed, they are transported to peripheral tissues for metabolism or are stored in reserve depots. The final common pathway for metabolism is the Krebs cycle, which utilizes acetyl-CoA for the point of entry.

in the process is converted to urea via the urea cycle in the liver (Conn and Stumpf, 1966). From this analysis, it can be seen that changes in body composition and organ function can have potentially important influences on energy homeostasis. Furthermore, BMR represents an overall assessment of many complex biochemical reactions, subcellular, cellular and organ interactions contributing to oxygen consumption and carbon dioxide production at rest. Thus, mechanisms which underlie changes in BMR can potentially act at many levels and be highly complex.

The regulatory processes which act to match food intake to energy requirements are poorly understood. The observation that body weight remains relatively constant for substantial periods of time indicates that short-term feeding behaviour and caloric intake must somehow be related to long-term caloric storage. The prevalence of obesity in affluent cultures indicates that such regulatory systems are frequently inadequate with resultant expansion of energy stores as fat.

Changes in food-seeking behaviour as well as in the process of food ingestion can influence this balance. The process of food intake is periodic. That is, food-seeking and ingestion begin at some point in time, continue for a finite period, and then stop. After an inter-meal period of variable length, food-seeking and ingestion begin again. The quantity of food ingested orally can be reduced by putting food in the stomach beforehand. However, the reduction in food intake is not sufficient to offset the caloric value of the food introduced into the stomach. Food is ingested most rapidly at the beginning of a meal with 50 per cent of the calories ingested in the initial 25 per cent of the feeding time (Bray, 1976). The composition of ingested nutrients depends on a complex interplay of psychological and gustatory influences determining taste preferences. Thus, changes in eating behaviour, psychological outlook, or taste perception may influence energy homeostasis in the elderly.

CHANGES OBSERVED WITH AGEING

While maladaptive psychological changes with ageing in man may impair the search for food and its subsequent intake, such changes are complex and difficult to document. However, objective changes in taste and smell have been observed which may directly decrease food intake or alter the types of foods which are selected. With ageing, there is a progressive loss in the number of taste buds per papilla on the tongue. The taste buds lost initially with ageing are on the anterior tongue, predominantly those detecting sweet and salty tastes. The taste buds remaining which detect primarily bitter or sour tastes thus show a relative increase with ageing, leading to a greater sensitivity to these gustatory sensations (Schiffman, 1973). In addition, the ability to identify foods while blindfolded decreases with advancing age (Schiffman, 1977). This is a commonly perceived problem among elderly individuals who complain of loss of both taste and smell (Cohen and Gitman, 1959). Thus, the choice of foods by the elderly may be changed as a result of decreased perceived food odour and a change in the taste of certain foods.

There are physical changes too diverse to catalogue here which make the mechanical processes of food preparation and eating more difficult for the elderly. For example, hand tremor, decreased visual acuity, decreased auditory acuity and the common use of dental plates all combine to make the social and physical components of eating more difficult (Barrows and Roeder, 1977). There are also changes in gastrointestinal function which can adversely affect food intake. There is a change in peristaltic activity of the oesophagus with ageing, termed presbyoesophagus (Bhanthumnavin and Schuster, 1977) which can result in a delay of oesophageal emptying.

Malabsorption and maldigestion exemplified by lactose intolerance can cause adverse symptoms after eating. Beyond these factors, the common occurrence of constipation with attendant laxative abuse and gaseous distension often affect the selection of foods (Bhanthumnavin and Schuster, 1977). Thus, elderly individuals may alter their food intake based on the expected effects of certain foods on gastrointestinal function.

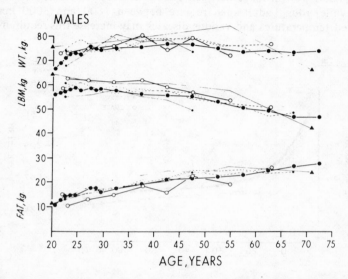

Fig. 1.3. Relation of age to body composition. These data for males show the changes in lean body mass and body fat from several studies. Note the rise in body weight early in adult life and the relative stability later on. In spite of the relative stability of body weight, fat as a percentage of the total rises progressively (Forbes and Reina, 1970).

Beyond the interactions of the elderly with their environment which influence nutrient intake, there are changes in body composition which may alter nutrient metabolism. Skeletal muscle mass represents a major store of protein calories and essential amino acids. This body compartment represents an important energy source during stress or early in starvation. Studies by Forbes and Reina (1970) using whole-body potassium levels as a determinant of muscle cell mass demonstrated a steady loss in lean body mass between the ages of 25 and 65 (*Fig.* 1.3). In addition, there was a steady increase in body fat in both males and females in adult life to age 85. During this period, body weight remained fairly constant. For instance, the Ten State Nutrition Survey (1972) documented a rise of 5 kg in average body weight of white males between ages 21 and 30. For white females there was a rise in body weight between ages 21 and 30, and a further rise to age 40. Thereafter, body weight remained fairly constant until age 70.

Changes in body weight and composition with age may be due in part to an imbalance between food intake and energy expenditure. Overall caloric requirements vary with age, sex, body weight and climate and are also influenced by drugs and hormones. The energy requirements of a young adult woman range between 1600 and 2200 kilocalories (kcal) per day, while young adult men require between 1800 and 3000 kcal/d. Elevated temperatures and various diseases may increase this requirement,

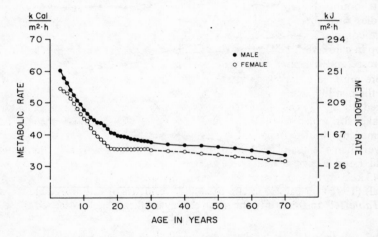

Fig. 1.4. Relation of metabolic rate to age. Males have a significantly higher metabolic rate at all ages than females. The decline in metabolism is rapid until age 20, but thereafter it slows.

while starvation reduces it (Bray, 1976). There are significant changes in energy requirements with ageing. At birth, total caloric needs are 120 kcal/kg, but these decline by 20 per cent during the first year of life. Over the next ten years, the requirement remains at about 80 kcal/kg until adolescence when they further decline to 50 kcal/kg in males and 35 kcal/kg in females. On an absolute basis, there is a gradual decline in energy requirements throughout the remainder of life as shown in *Fig.* 1.4. When corrected for the rising surface area during growth, however, energy requirements decline little during this period. The fall is most rapid during childhood. Between age 18 and 20, the rate of decline levels off, and in adult life, drops by between 2 and 5 per cent per decade. For the reference man who is 22 years old and weighs 67 kg, the caloric requirements are set at 3000 kcal or approximately 45 kcal/kg. For the reference female who is 22 years old and weighs 48 kg, the requirements are 2200 kcal or

36 kcal/kg (Recommended Dietary Allowances, 1978). These caloric requirements decline by approximately 5 per cent per decade between age 20 and 35, and by 2—3 per cent per decade for the next 20 years.

Estimation of caloric intake can be done in a variety of ways. It can be done using a method of 24-hour recall, or by using a 3-day recall method. It can also be done with a diary and a notebook method. In normal weight adults these methods are thought to be within 10 per cent of the true intakes. However, the correlation between caloric intake from day to day and the expenditure of energy is low. The poor correlation between observed intake of food and the energy expenditure of military recruits casts doubts on all short-term measurements, yet for most population studies such measurements are all that we have. McGandy et al. (1966) have compared the dietary records for 252 men aged 20—99. There was a drop in caloric intake which averaged 12·4 cal per day for each year of age increase and a decline in metabolic rate of 5·23 cal/d/year, indicating that there must be a decline in energy expenditure related to physical activity. In their study, men aged 20—34 took in an average of 2688 kcal/d compared to 2093 kcal/d for men aged 75—99 years. Estimates of caloric intake for males from the Household Food Consumption Survey performed by the US Department of Agriculture in 1965—66 were somewhat lower than the figures obtained by McGandy et al. (1966). In the Household Food Consumption Survey, caloric intake of men aged 35—54 was 2643 kcal/d. For men over 75 it was 1866 kcal/d. The data from Lonergan et al. (1975) on caloric intake of elderly residents of Edinburgh are shown in *Table* 1.1. In this study the mean energy intakes in men exceeded those in

Table 1.1. Daily caloric intake of elderly males and females from Edinburgh

Age	Males (N)	Females (N)
	kcal/d	
62—74	2494 (158)	1771 (190)
75—90	2176 (54)	1648 (73)

women, and in both sexes energy intake decreased with age. The most extensive survey known to the authors on caloric intake in relation to age is that compiled by the National Center for Health Statistics as part of the Health and Nutrition Examination Survey (HANES) conducted between 1971 and 1974. These data for males and females over age 20 are summarized in *Table* 1.2. Until age 45 the men are consuming on average 1000 kcal/d more than the women, and even in the population aged 65—74 the men still had an intake nearly 500 kcal/d more than the women. The relatively low levels of energy intake for many women in this survey suggest that the dietary standards for WHO/FAO, for the National Academy of Sciences,

Table 1.2. Estimated caloric intake in relation to age

Age	Sex			
	Males		Females	
	N	kcal/d	N	kcal/d
20–24	513	2888	1243	1691
25–34	804	2739	1896	1638
35–44	665	2554	1663	1558
45–54	765	2301	836	1533
55–64	597	2076	670	1382
65–74	1657	1805	1822	1307

US National Center for Health Statistics [DHEW (MRA) 77–1647].
Dietary Intake Findings United States 1971–74.

National Research Council and for the Canadian Recommended Dietary Allowances are too high. Indeed these guidelines for energy intake should probably be expressed as a range of generally acceptable intakes since the variables of size, activity and metabolism cannot allow a single figure to apply to a whole population.

DuBois (1936) noted a large variation in the basal metabolic rate (BMR) of older people and thought this might be dependent upon some element of senility. In one study of 17 older females aged 60–69, Durnin (1959) found a caloric requirement of 1900 kcal/d. Matson and Hitchcock (1934) studied 8 females aged 77–106, and 17 males aged 74–92, and found heat production of 1046 kcal/d for the females and 1210 kcal/d for the males. They noted that these values were considerably below the standard for metabolic rate published by Aub and DuBois (1917). In one careful longitudinal study, Magnus-Levy (1942) reported his own metabolic rate to be 231 ml of oxygen per minute at age 26, and that it had declined to a figure of 176 ml/min by age 76, a decline of 24 per cent during this 50-year period.

The decreases observed with ageing in overall metabolic rate may reflect decreases in many of the metabolic components involved in energy homeostasis. For example, serum cholesterol levels appear to show a general increase with age (Lopez et al., 1967; Werner et al., 1970). A recent study of men and women in London (Slack et al., 1977) demonstrated an increase in cholesterol levels in men from 214 mg/dl at 30–39 years of age to 233 mg/dl at 40–49 years of age, with relatively stable levels thereafter. Levels of cholesterol in women rise later, but ultimately reach levels higher than those found in men in the 50–59 year age group (Slack et al., 1977). Studies in ageing rats (Kritchevsky, 1972a) have shown that cholesterol turnover, synthesis, and degradation rates are all decreased progressively with age. Whether similar changes occur in humans with ageing has not yet been determined. However, increased deposition of esterified cholesterol in the aorta with age has been demonstrated (Kritchevsky, 1972b), and may reflect a decrease in the rate of exchange of cholesterol between the rapidly exchanging pools of cholesterol in the body and the more slowly exchangeable forms deposited in tissues, where they may promote atherogenesis (Smith, 1965). In additon, rates of whole-body protein turnover progressively decrease with age (Munro and Young, 1978), and this decrease may significantly contribute to the overall decrease in metabolic rate. Impaired glucose tolerance often occurs in the elderly, but whether this is due to decreased physical activity, decreased pancreatic function, or a slowing in glucose-metabolic processes is unknown. Changes in other components of the BMR such as ion pumping have not been studied. Nonetheless, metabolic changes secondary to decreased metabolite turnover with ageing may contribute to the changes in body fat and muscle cell mass observed in the elderly.

DIETARY GUIDELINES FOR THE ELDERLY
General dietary guidelines for the elderly can be developed based on the principles of energy homeostasis already outlined and the changes in energy homeostasis observed with ageing. First, food intake should match

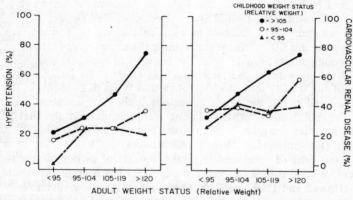

Fig. 1.5. Relation of weight in childhood and weight in adult life to the prevalence of hypertension and cardiovascular renal disease. The individuals who gained weight in adult life and who were of normal weight or less in childhood showed the highest incidence of both diseases (Abraham et al., 1971).

energy expenditure. As physical activity and the rate of metabolic processes decrease with ageing, energy intake should be reduced. Excess energy intake with ageing commonly leads to increased body fat which offsets decreased muscle mass to keep body weight relatively constant. Obesity is known to be a risk factor for the development of cardiovascular disease, renal disease and hypertension. Abraham et al. (1971) reported on 717 white males examined at ages 9–13 between 1923 and 1928, and subsequently examined at an average age of 48. As shown in *Fig.* 1.5, individuals who moved from below to average weight between childhood and adult life had a substantially higher prevalence of hypertension and renal vascular disease than those who remained at their initial relative weight status. In the Framingham Study (Kannel, 1973), an increase of 50 per cent in ideal body weight in men led to a 100 per cent increased risk of cardiovascular disorders. Both hypertension and hypercholesterolaemia, the most prominent risk factors for cardiovascular disease, are aggravated by increasing weight status. Whether the relative increase in body fat with ageing has similar implications is unclear, but studies of longevity show some advantage for individuals with below average weight (Bray et al., 1972). Second, sufficient essential nutrients, vitamins and minerals must be supplied whenever an effort is made to restrict total energy intake. Altered food selection by the elderly based on the psychological and physiological changes already outlined may contribute to the well-documented increased incidence of multiple vitamin deficiencies in the elderly population as a whole (Marks, 1969). Energy restriction, if not carefully planned, could result in aggravation of these deficiencies and the occurrence of protein, essential fatty acid and mineral deficiencies. The Food and Nutrition Board of the National Academy of Science/National Research Council of the United States (Recommended Dietary Allowances, 1974), recommends a decrease in total caloric intake in both men and women after age 50, while recommending the same level of vitamin intake as for young adults aged 19—22. The benefits of multivitamin therapy in the elderly are evident, but attention also needs to be directed at assessments of the quality and quantity of various types of nutrients in the diet to be assured that basic needs in various body compartments are being met. The Food and Nutrition Board recommends that the diet of the elderly includes 0·6 g/kg of high quality protein or 0·8 g/kg of mixed proteins (Recommended Dietary Allowances, 1979). A diet in which 50—55 per cent of total caloric intake consists of carbohydrates and 30 per cent of total calories is contributed by fat has been recommended by some (Howell and Loeb, 1969) but may not be generally advisable. Within these two food groups, starches and polyunsaturated fats are preferred by some to sugar and saturated fats respectively, but these considerations are outside the scope of this chapter. Finally, dietary guidelines for the elderly must incorporate some consideration of the physical and psychological aspects of food ingestion. Their altered tastes specifically change the palatability of many foods commonly eaten by younger individuals. Altered gastrointestinal function necessitates the addition and elimination of specific types of food. Thus, pragmatic dietary research must be done to promote the compliance of elderly individuals with diets incorporating recommended changes in energy and nutrient intake.

Elderly populations are growing rapidly in affluent cultures as modern medicine and better living standards reduce or eliminate many of the illnesses which caused premature deaths in the past. However, chronic diseases and decreasing quality of life among the elderly have become an increasingly evident problem. While some factors influencing health, such as hereditary predisposition to disease, are beyond the control of the individual, improved nutrition is an attainable goal that would be likely to improve the quality of life among the elderly. Finally, basic and applied research in this important area is needed to improve the nutritional and energy intake of the elderly.

REFERENCES

Abraham S., Collins G. and Nordsieck M. (1971) *HSMHA Health Reports* **86**, 273.
Anderson W. F. (1974) *J. Am. Geriatr. Soc.* **22**, 385.
Aub J. C. and DuBois E. F. (1917) *Arch. Intern. Med.* **19**, 823.
Barrows C. H. and Roeder L. M. (1977) In: Finch C. and Hayflick L. (ed.), *The Handbook of the Biology of Aging*. New York, Van Nostrand Reinhold, p. 561.
Bhanthumnavin K. and Schuster M. D. (1977) In: Finch C. and Hayflick L. (ed.), *The Handbook of the Biology of Aging*. New York, Van Nostrand Reinhold, p. 709.
Bray G. A. (1976) In: *The Obese Patient*. Philadelphia, Saunders.
Bray G. A., Davidson M. B. and Drenick E. J. (1972) *Ann. Intern. Med.* **77**, 779.
Chope H. D. and Breslow L. (1956) *Am. J. Public Health* **46**, 61.
Cohen T. and Gitman L. (1959) *J. Gerontol.* **14**, 294.
Conn E. E. and Stumpf P. K. (1966) *Outlines of Biochemistry*. New York, Wiley, p. 346.
Consolazio C. F., Johnson R. E. and Pecora L. J. (1963) *Physiological Measurements of Metabolic Function in Man*. New York, McGraw-Hill, p. 1.
Dreizen S. (1974) *Geriatrics* **24**, 97.
DuBois E. F. (1936) *Basal Metabolism in Health Disease*. Philadelphia, Lea & Febiger.
Durnin J. V. G. A. (1959) *Br. J. Nutr.* **13**, 68.
Eckstein D. (1973) *J. Am. Geriatr. Soc.* **21**, 440.
Forbes G. B. and Reina J. C. (1970) *Metabolism* **19**, 653.
Howell S. C. and Loeb M. B. (1969) *Gerontologist* Autumn, 17.
Kannel W. B. (1973) *Nutr. Am. Heart* **1**, 104.
Kaplan L., Landes J. H. and Pincus J. (1955) *Geriatrics* **10**, 287.
Kritchevsky D. (1972a) *Mech. Ageing Dev.* **1**, 275.
Kritchevsky D. (1972b) *Lipids* **7**, 305.
Lonergan M. E., Milne J. S., Maule M. M. et al. (1975) *Br. J. Nutr.* **34**, 517.
Lopez S. A., Kreshl W. A. and Hodges R. E. (1967) *Am. J. Clin. Nutr.* **20**, 808.
McGandy R. B., Burrows C. H., Spanias A. et al. (1966) *J. Gerontol.* **21**, 581.
Magnus-Levy A. (1942) *J. Am. Med. Assoc.* **118**, 1369.
Marks J. (1969) *R. Soc. Health J.* **87**, 289.
Matson J. R. and Hitchcock F. A. (1934) *Am. J. Physiol.* **110**, 329.
Moore F. D. and Brennan M. F. (1974) In: Ballinger W. F. (ed.), *Manual of Surgical Nutrition*. Philadelphia, Saunders, p. 109.
Munro H. N. and Young V. R. (1978) *Postgrad. Med.* **63**, 143.
NAS/NRC (1974; 1978; 1979) (*see* General References.)
Schiffman S. S. (1973) In: Busse E. W. and Pfeiffer E. (ed.), *Mental Illness in Later Life*. American Psychiatric Association, p. 269.
Schiffman S. S. (1977) *J. Gerontol.* **5**, 586.
Slack J., Noble N. and Meade T. W. (1977) *Br. Med. J.* **2**, 353.
Smith E. B. (1965) *J. Atherosclerosis* **5**, 224.
Steinkamp R. C., Cohen N. L. and Walsh H. E. (1965) *J. Am. Diet. Assoc.* **46**, 103.

Ten State Nutrition Survey (1972) US DHEW Publication (HSM) 72−8131. US Department of Agriculture (1966) Household Food Consumption Survey (1965−66).

US National Center for Health Statistics *Dietary Intake Findings, United States, 1971−74.* DHEW (MRA) 77−1647.

Werner M., Rolls R. E. and Hultin J. V. (1970) *J. Clin. Chem. Clin. Biochem.* 8, 105.

WHO/FAO (1973) *(see* General References.)

2. PROTEIN METABOLISM AND REQUIREMENTS
H. N. Munro and V. R. Young

People who have ceased to grow because they are adults do not cease to undergo changes which take the form of alterations in body composition and tissue structure. This is well-established in the case of fat deposition, but there are less obvious changes in the amount of active tissues such as muscle, and in the functional capacity of organs such as the kidney, which are progressive throughout adult life. In consequence, some indices such as renal function and maximum oxygen uptake at 75 years of age can be less than 50 per cent of their capacity at 25 years. This short review will evaluate changes in whole-body protein metabolism during ageing and will relate this to the needs of the elderly for dietary protein. Further discussion of this area is available in recent reviews (Young et al., 1976a, b; Uauy et al., 1978c).

PROTEIN METABOLISM
Body Composition and Muscle Mass
Ageing is accompanied by changes in the amount and distribution of protein within the body. Using whole-body potassium as an index of body protein content, both cross-sectional (Allen et al., 1960; Forbes and Reina 1970; Parizkova et al., 1971) and longitudinal studies (Forbes and Reina, 1970) show that there is a reduction in the amount of total body protein with advancing age in both men and women (*Fig.* 2.1). The contribution made by each of the body organs to the loss of body protein content is not precisely known, but *Fig.* 2.2, based on dissection at autopsy (Korenchevsky, 1961), shows that a major proportion of this loss is due to a reduction in skeletal muscle mass. At the time of birth, muscle accounts for some 25 per cent of body weight, increasing to 45 per cent in the young adult and then declining to 27 per cent beyond age 70. In contrast, the liver contributes a progressively smaller proportion of body weight from birth onwards, so that it declines from 4 per cent at birth to about 3 per cent in the young adult and 2 per cent in the elderly.

Further support for these changing ratios comes from studies of the relationship between creatinine excretion and lean body mass. The output of urinary creatinine is assumed to be a measure of muscle mass, especially when dietary intake of creatine is low, as in the case of subjects on a

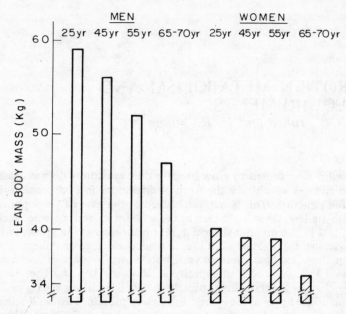

Fig. 2.1. Mean values for lean body mass (from ^{40}K) at selected ages in men and women. (*Drawn from data of Forbes and Reina, 1970.*)

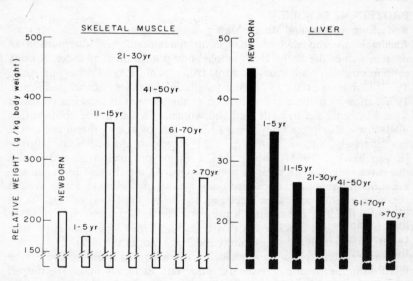

Fig. 2.2. Relative weights of skeletal muscle and liver at various ages in human subjects. (*Drawn from tabular data of Korenchevsky, 1961.*)

synthetic formula diet. Elderly subjects show a lower creatinine output per unit of body weight, which shares the reduction in their lower body cell mass, as determined from whole-body ^{40}K (Uauy et al., 1978d). Since skeletal muscle is such a large proportion of total body protein and makes adaptations under various dietary, hormonal and stressful conditions (Young, 1970), it is desirable to assess the quantitative contribution of skeletal muscle to whole-body protein metabolism in elderly subjects. We shall therefore examine the effect of ageing on turnover of whole-body muscle protein.

Turnover of Body Protein

The changes in the relative proportions of various organs during growth, development and subsequent ageing are accompanied by significant alterations in the dynamics of metabolism. *Table* 2.1 summarizes pub-

Table 2.1. Rates of whole-body protein synthesis at various ages

Group	Age or weight	Number in group	Method	Protein synthesis (g/kg/d)	Reference
Premature infants	1—45 days	5	^{15}N-glycine infusion	26·3	Pencharz et al. (1977)
	42—68 days	3	^{15}N-glycine orally	10·0—15·5	Nicholson, (1970)
Infants	5 kg	3	^{15}N-aspartate orally	3·3—7·7	Wu and Snyderman (1959)
	10—20 months	5	^{15}N-glycine infusion	6·1	Picou and Taylor-Roberts (1969)
Children	9—16 years	8	^{15}N-glycine infusion	3·7	Kien et al. (1978)
Young Adults:					
Males			^{15}N-glycine infusion	3·3	Uauy et al. (1978d)
Females			^{15}N-glycine infusion	2·6	Uauy et al. (1978d)
Elderly:					
Males			^{15}N-glycine infusion	2·9	Uauy et al. (1978d)
Females			^{15}N-glycine infusion	2·3	Uauy et al. (1978d)

lished estimates of the rates of body protein synthesis at different stages in life. During growth and development, the rate of whole-body protein turnover (synthesis and breakdown) falls as adulthood approaches and then continues to decline more slowly during the adult years. It will be noted (*Table* 2.1) that synthesis per kg body weight is less in adult women than men, but both sexes show a significant decline with age. Recently, we (Uauy et al., 1978d) have compared rates of synthesis and of breakdown of whole-body protein in elderly human subjects of both sexes. *Table* 2.2 summarizes these studies and shows that breakdown as well as synthesis follows the same pattern of reduction during ageing.

It has also been shown that the effects of advancing years in the adult are to cause redistribution of protein metabolism so that the musculature provides a progressively decreasing proportion of total protein metabolism (Uauy et al., 1978d). The impact of the reduced muscle mass on the contribution of muscle to whole-body protein turnover can be explored by estimating rates of muscle protein breakdown compared with those of whole-body protein breakdown. This can be achieved through the use

Table 2.2. Rates of synthesis and breakdown of protein by the whole body in young adults and elderly subjects (from Uauy et al., 1978d)

| Group | Whole-body protein | | | |
| | Synthesis | | Breakdown | |
	g/d	g/kg	g/d	g/kg/d
Young adult				
Male	255±39	3·33±0·3	255±31	2·94±0·2
Female	157±18	2·63±0·2	142±20	2·35±0·1
Elderly				
Male	202±26	2·94±0·7	181±25	2·64±0·7
Female	123±28	2·25±0·4	106±27	1·94±0·4
$F_{(13, 16)}$[a]	18·44	3·86	17·69	3·82
P	<0·01	<0·05	<0·01	<0·05

[a] F ratio. For statistical significance by analysis of variance.

of urinary N^{γ}-methylhistidine (3-methylhistidine) excretion. Elsewhere, we (Young et al., 1973; Young and Munro, 1978) have reviewed the evidence indicating that the output of this amino acid gives a quantitative index of the breakdown of muscle protein *in vivo* in rats and human subjects. Thus, the determination of muscle protein breakdown rate by this means involves the following considerations: (*a*) the major site of the amino acid 3-methylhistidine is in the myofibrillar proteins of skeletal muscle, namely actin and myosin; (*b*) this amino acid is formed in these proteins by methylation of a histidine residue after peptide bond synthesis; (*c*) upon breakdown of actin and myosin, the amino acid is released and quantitatively excreted in the urine, without undergoing significant metabolic alterations in man (Long et al., 1974) or the rat (Young et al., 1972). Thus, daily excretion of 3-methylhistidine is related quantitatively to its release from the major myofibrillar proteins in skeletal muscle, and in consequence reflects the rate of breakdown of these proteins.

Accordingly, the urinary excretion of 3-methylhistidine was measured in young adults and elderly subjects consuming flesh-free diets. The use of such diets is to avoid exogenous sources of 3-methylhistidine. Assuming a concentration of 4·2 μmol 3-methylhistidine per gram mixed protein (Bilmazes et al., 1978), *Fig.* 2.3 shows that muscle breakdown accounts for approximately 27 per cent of whole-body protein breakdown in young adults. For the elderly, on the other hand, muscle accounts for a significantly lower proportion of whole-body protein breakdown; in this case the mean values were 16 per cent and 20 per cent for elderly women and men,

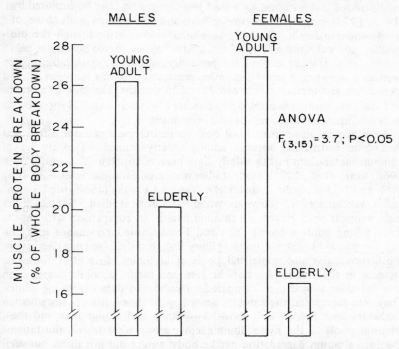

Fig. 2.3. Comparison of the contribution of skeletal muscle to whole-body protein breakdown in young adults and elderly subjects. (*Taken from Uauy et al., 1978d.*)

respectively (Uauy et al., 1978d). Thus, there is a shift in favour of visceral protein turnover in the elderly adult.

Few other tissue proteins have been studied metabolically in relation to ageing in human subjects. However, some data on albumin metabolism has been obtained in both ageing animals and ageing man. Old rats, as compared to young rats, have been noted to synthesize albumin at greater rates *in vivo* (Beauchenne et al., 1970). Chen et al. (1973) demonstrated that albumin synthesis from isolated liver microsomes is 50 per cent higher than that of young rats, whereas there was no difference in total liver protein synthesis. Obenrader et al. (1975) isolated mRNA (messenger ribonucleic acid) from old and young rats and determined that there was significantly more total mRNA isolated from old rat liver polysomes, but that the increased total mRNA was entirely due to albumin mRNA. Chen et al. (1973) also observed that young rats increased albumin synthesis by 40 per cent in response to bleeding whereas old rats showed no increase in albumin synthesis under these conditions. They suggested that the rate of albumin synthesis in old rats is maximal and therefore does not respond to the added stress caused by blood loss. Recently, Van Benzooijen et al. (1976; 1977) measured protein synthesis and albumin synthesis in isolated rat parenchymal cells. The cells were incubated in a modified Waymouth medium and achieved a level of albumin synthesis approximately equal to *in vivo* rates. The capacity of the parenchymal cells to synthesize protein decreased between 3 and 12 months, remained constant between 12 and 24 months, and increased between 24 and 35 months. The ratio of albumin to total liver protein was relatively constant between 3 and 24 months but increased markedly between 24 and 36 months.

Low plasma albumin without obvious pathological cause is a frequent finding in nutritional surveys among elderly humans. Two studies of albumin metabolism in the elderly have been conducted (Yan and Franks, 1968; Misra et al., 1975). Both studies measured catabolic rates only using ^{131}I- and ^{125}I-albumin, respectively. Yan and Franks (1968) used 3 men and 3 women aged 72–85 years, while Misra et al. studied 9 females and 5 male subjects aged 70–86, all in good health. In comparison with results from young adult subjects, Yan and Franks noted no change in extravascular passage times and transcapillary flux, but did observe a decrease in the intravascular and interstitial pools of albumin. Misra et al. found an increase in the fractional catabolic rate and in the absolute degradation rate for their subjects, as compared to published data on young adults. They also segregated the subjects according to those with plasma albumin concentrations below and above 3 g/100ml and found that, although albumin pools in the hypo-albuminaemic group were lower, the rate of absolute albumin degradation per kg body weight did not differ between the groups. Accordingly, the resultant turnover represented a higher proportion of the albumin pool of the hypo-albuminaemic group. Consequently, the authors postulate an impairment in the control of degradation among the elderly. Methodologically, both of these studies have serious limitations. Since plasma albumin concentration is commonly used as a biochemical index of protein nutritional status, the occurrence of changes in albumin metabolism with advancing age needs to be more fully explored.

Recent studies of albumin turnover in elderly adults performed in our laboratory show that albumin metabolism in the elderly is *not* accelerated at an adequate level of protein intake. The rate of albumin synthesis was obtained by modifying the procedure of McFarlane (1964), in which ^{14}C-labelling of urea provided a measure of the ^{14}C specific activity of the guanidino carbon of arginine and thus of liver-free arginine, the precursor of arginine in newly synthesized plasma albumin. In our studies, the stable isotope ^{15}N was administered in the form of ^{15}N-glycine continuously over several days to healthy elderly subjects and the appearance of ^{15}N in arginine of plasma albumin and in urinary urea was used to calculate albumin synthesis rate from the precursor pool of arginine in the liver. On an adequate intake of protein, the fractional rate of synthesis and the total rate of synthesis (fractional rate $\times$ plasma albumin content) were less than in young adults. When the young subjects were fed a diet low in protein for 14 days, they responded with a reduction in rate of albumin synthesis, but the rate remained unchanged when the old subjects received a similar low-protein diet. Thus the rate of albumin synthesis in the young, but not the elderly, is responsive to changes in protein intake. It may be that maximum albumin synthesis is controlled by a set-point, which prevents responses to increased protein intakes, and that this set-point is much lower in old people, thus limiting their response to dietary protein.

Protein Needs and Allowances

The protein requirements of adult men and women have been estimated by a number of investigators, mostly studying young adult populations. The elderly are generally less accessible, and can suffer from chronic disease that is likely to affect protein needs. In the past, protein requirements have been estimated by a factorial method which includes measurements of the output of nitrogen by subjects on a protein-free diet (obligatory N loss) and estimates of the amounts of dietary protein needed to prevent such N losses from causing a negative N balance. Each of these will be considered and finally our knowledge of the effects of various diseases on the need for dietary protein will be summarized.

1. Obligatory Nitrogen Losses and Estimated Protein Requirements

Scrimshaw et al. (1976) and Uauy et al. (1978a) measured the obligatory urinary and faecal nitrogen losses in elderly men and women after the subjects had adapted to a short period on a diet low in protein. Urinary nitrogen excretion fell with ingestion of the protein-free diet and the pattern of change in daily nitrogen output was similar to that in young adults (*Fig.* 2.4). These data provide the basis for estimating the protein requirements of adults of various ages according to the factorial method (WHO/FAO, 1973) as described in *Table* 2.3. Thus, the factorial estimate for elderly subjects is shown in the table, and is compared with values for young adults under similar dietary conditions. By this method the reference protein (egg or milk) allowances for elderly men and women are no greater and indeed somewhat less than those for young adults. A number of assumptions are made, however, in arriving at the estimations given in *Table* 2.3. First it is assumed that the efficiency of dietary nitrogen utilization at requirement levels is the same in young and elderly adults.

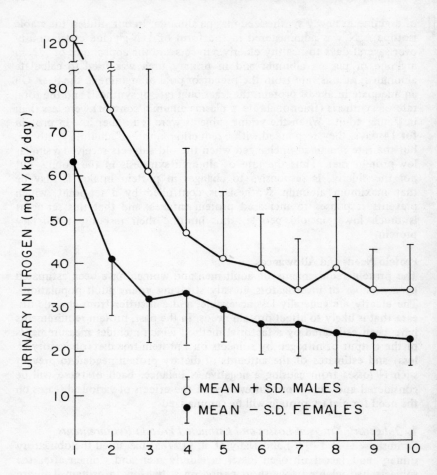

Fig. 2.4. Change in urinary nitrogen excretion in elderly men and women during use of protein-free diet. (*Taken from Uauy et al., 1978a.*)

Second, the extent of variability in nitrogen requirements among apparently similar subjects is taken to be the same in elderly and young adults. Third, in the conversion of the allowance for egg or milk protein to protein of lower quality, it is assumed that the relative differences in nutritional value of protein foods are the same in healthy young and elderly adults. There are insufficient data to assess the validity of each of these three assumptions and accordingly direct nitrogen balance studies designed to determine the minimum physiological requirements for nitrogen are considered in the following section.

Table 2.3. Factorial determination of protein requirement of various adult groups (from Uauy et al., 1978a)

Group	Mean total obligatory nitrogen loss (mg/kg/d)	Adjusted mean nitrogen requirement (mg/kg/d)[a]	Safe levels of intake [b]	
			Nitrogen (mg/kg/d)	Protein (g/kg/d)[c]
Men	54	70	91	0·57
Women	49	64	83	0·52
Elderly				
Women	39	51	67	0·42
Men	52	67	87	0·55

[a] Obligatory nitrogen losses are increased by 30 per cent to account for efficiency of nitrogen utilization.

[b] Values are adjusted requirements plus 30 per cent to allow for individual variability.

[c] As egg or milk protein.
Data for men and women WHO/FAO (1973).

2. Nitrogen Balance Studies

Direct determination of the requirement for protein in elderly subjects depends upon reliable nitrogen balance information in the near-maintenance region of total nitrogen intake. Published nitrogen balance studies in elderly subjects have been reviewed by us and by others and show that the results are too variable to permit definitive conclusions regarding the minimum protein needs of older people. The reasons for the discrepancies include differences in experimental approach and in the nutritional and health status of the subjects used in these studies, as well as inability to assess minimum levels of protein intake for nitrogen equilibrium.

We (Uauy et al., 1978c) have carried out studies in a group of healthy elderly men and women to obtain the nitrogen balance response to graded intakes of good quality protein, with the objective of identifying minimum levels of high quality protein sufficient to maintain nitrogen equilibrium. The results of two such series of studies, involving men and women, are shown in *Fig.* 2.5. It is apparent from these that the nitrogen requirement of nearly all elderly subjects receiving a high quality food protein cannot be met at the intake level that is predicted by the factorial method. For example, this latter approach suggested that the allowance for elderly women would be 0·42 g/kg per day whereas the nitrogen balance data shown in *Fig.* 2.5 indicate that this level of intake would not be adequate. The reason for this large discrepancy is not clear, but it includes underestimation of one or both factors used in adjusting mean values of total obligatory nitrogen losses to arrive at the population requirement. For a mixed diet, the allowance of protein for adults recommended in the RDA for the U.S. (NAS/NRC, 1980) is 0·8 g protein/kg per day. However, Cheng et al. (1978) found that an intake of 0·8 g protein/kg from a mixture of wheat-soy-milk maintained N balance in only four out of seven elderly male subjects.

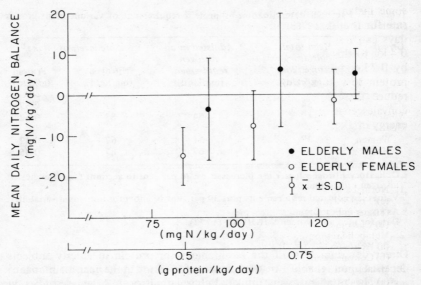

Fig. 2.5. Nitrogen balance in 8 elderly males and 7 elderly females on graded levels of egg protein intake. (*From data of Uauy et al., 1978c.*)

In attempting to utilize the results of the above studies to arrive at dietary protein allowances, it is important to recognize that there are numerous factors that modify the nutrient needs of individuals and population groups, some of which are discussed below. This makes the formulation of an appropriate or safe dietary protein allowance for the elderly population particularly difficult. Until more data become available, we conclude that diets of the elderly should supply more than 10 per cent of the calories as protein and that a holistic estimate is probably 12—14 per cent.

PROTEIN REQUIREMENTS IN DISEASE

As age progresses, there is an increasing incidence of serious disease. Some chronic diseases cause impaired utilization of dietary protein, others result in temporary losses of body protein that have to be restored during convalescence. Consequently, the elderly can quite frequently have an increased need for protein.

Changes in protein needs in disease are difficult to assess, since diseases vary in their intensity. Accordingly, *Table* 2.4 provides only rough estimates of the orders of magnitude of changes in protein and energy needs in some major diseases. Conditions resulting in losses of body protein include fever, injury (including notably burns) and planned operations. The degree of body protein loss varies considerably, and can in some instances double the dietary needs for protein in order to compensate for the loss. Thus simple disuse atrophy from rest in bed over several days can result in a loss of 0·3 kg body protein, while gastrectomy adds 0·4 kg to this loss of body protein, fracture of a femur increases the loss by 0·7 kg and a 35 per cent burn can add 1·2 kg to the amount of body protein lost as a result of bed rest (Cuthbertson, 1972). Attempts to reduce these losses during the acute phase and to replace them during convalescence have led to recommendations for increased protein and energy intakes (*Table* 2.4).

Table 2.4. Protein requirements in specific diseases (from Munro, 1977)

1. Normal adult:—
   (a) For N equilibrium: 0·6 g/kg raised to 0·8 g/kg by protein quality correction (80 per cent).
   (b) Customary intake: 1—2 g/kg
2. Metabolic response to severe injury and burning:—
   (a) Acute phase: 2 + g/kg + cals
   (b) Convalescence: 2 + g/kg
3. Malabsorption and gastrointestinal diseases:—
   (a) Malabsorption syndrome: 1 g/kg
   (b) Ulcerative colitis: 1—1·4 g/kg†
   (c) Ileocaecostomy: 1—1·4 g/kg†
4. Liver disease:—
   (a) Acute hepatic encephalopathy: very low*
   (b) Recovered encephalopathy: 1—1·5 g/kg
   (c) Chronic encephalopathy: 0·5 g/kg*
5. Renal disease:—
   (a) Uraemia: 0·5 g/kg*
   (b) Nephrosis: 1—1·4 g/kg†
6. Malignant disease:—
   Increased protein and energy

*Intake restricted on clinical grounds.
†In each condition, losses of protein can double minimal requirements.

The cachexia of malignant disease is a special form of body protein loss accompanied by other metabolic changes and by anorexia (Goodlad, 1964; Munro, 1977). Recent studies (Copeland et al., 1977) show that the malnutrition of the cachectic cancer case causes loss of cellular immunological responses which can be restored by vigorous nutritional measures including parenteral nutrition. These changes, and the accompanying restoration of tissue function, have important consequences for the patient. An extensive series of cases treated in this way by Copeland et al. (1977) shows that the prognoses for operation, irradiation and chemotherapy are much improved by realimentation.

Increased need for protein can occur as a result of gastrointestinal disease leading to less efficient absorption, or increased losses of protein

(*Table* 2.4). Finally, chronic liver or renal failure requires careful restriction of protein intake in order not to overload these organs (*Table* 2.4).

CONCLUSIONS

Progressive loss of body protein is a major feature of ageing throughout adult life. This appears to affect some tissues, notably muscle, more than others. There is no direct evidence to suggest that this erosion of tissue protein is due to lack of adequate amounts of protein in the average diet. Nevertheless, there are some data showing that many older people, especially those with chronic diseases, may require more protein than do young adults in order to achieve nitrogen equilibrium. Since caloric intake declines progressively with ageing (McGandy et al., 1966), this implies that an increasingly larger percentage of dietary energy intake should consist of protein in order to maintain nitrogen balance. The significance of this for selection by the elderly of diets with a higher than average protein concentration deserves investigation.

REFERENCES

Allen T. H., Anderson E. C. and Langham W. H. (1960) *J. Gerontol.* 15, 348.
Beauchenne R. E., Roeder L. M. and Barrows C. H. jun. (1970) *J. Gerontol.* 25, 359.
Bilmazes C., Uauy R., Haverberg L. N. et al. (1978) *Metabolism* 27, 525.
Chen J. C., Ove P. and Lansing A. J. (1973) *Biochim. Biophys. Acta* 312, 598.
Cheng A. H. R., Gomez A., Bergan J. G. et al. (1978) *Am. J. Clin. Nutr.* 31, 12.
Copeland E. M., Daly J. M. and Dudrick S. J. (1977) *Cancer Res.* 37, 2451.
Cuthbertson D. P. (1972) In: Wilkinson A. W. (ed.), *Parenteral Nutrition.* London, Churchill, pp. 4–15.
Forbes G. B. and Reina J. C. (1970) *Metabolism* 19, 653.
Goodlad G. A. J. (1964) In: Munro H. N. and Allison J. B. (ed.), *Mammalian Protein Metabolism*, Vol. 2., New York, Academic, p. 415.
Kien C. L., Rohrbaugh D. K., Burke J. F. et al. (1978) *Pediatr. Res.* 12, 211.
Korenchevsky V. (1961) In: Bourne G. H. (ed.), *Physiological and Pathological Ageing.* New York, Hafner, p. 541.
Long C. L., Haverberg L. N., Young V. R. et al. (1974) *Metabolism* 24, 929.
McFarlane A. S. (1964) *Biochem. J.* 89, 277.
McGandy R. B., Barrows C. H. jun., Spanias A. et al. (1966) *J. Gerontol.* 21, 581.
Misra D. P., Loudon J. M. and Staddan G. E. (1975) *J. Gerontol.* 30, 304.
Munro H. N. (1977) *J. Am. Diet. Assoc.* 71, 380.
NAS/NRC (1980) (*see* General References).
Nicholson J. F. (1970) *Ped. Res.* 4, 389.
Obenrader M., Chen J., Ove P. et al. (1975) In: Cristofalo V. J., Roberts J. and Adelman R. C. (ed.), *Exploration in Aging.* New York, Plenum, pp. 289–290.
Parizkova J., Eiselt E., Sprynarova S. et al. (1971) *J. Appl. Physiol.* 31, 323.
Pencharz P. B., Steffe W. P., Cochran W. et al. (1977) *Clin. Sci. Mol. Med.* 52, 485.
Picou D. and Taylor-Roberts T. (1969) *Clin. Sci.* 36, 283.
Scrimshaw N. S., Perera W. D. A. and Young V. R. (1976) *J. Nutr.* 106, 665.
Uauy R., Scrimshaw N. S., Rand W. M. et al. (1978a) *J. Nutr.* 108, 97.
Uauy R., Scrimshaw N. S. and Young V. R. (1978b) In: *Nutrition of the Aged. Symp. Proc. Nutr. Soc. Canada*, Quebec, pp. 53–71.
Uauy R., Scrimshaw N. S. and Young V. R. (1978c) *Am. J. Clin. Nutr.* 31, 779.
Uauy R., Winterer J. C., Bilmazes C. et al. (1978d) *J. Gerontol.* 33, 663.

Van Benzooijen F., Grell T. and Knook D. L. (1976) *Biochem. Biophys. Res. Commun.* 71, 513.

Van Benzooijen F., Grell T. and Knook D. L. (1977) *Mech. Aging Dev.* 6, 293.

WHO/FAO (1973) (*see* General References).

Wu H. and Snyderman S. E. (1959) *J. Gen. Physiol.* 34, 339.

Yas S. H. Y. and Franks J. J. (1968) *J. Lab. Clin. Med.* 72, 449.

Young V. R. (1970) In: Munro H. N. (ed.), *Mammalian Protein Metabolism*, Vol. IV. New York, Academic, pp. 585–674.

Young V. R., Alexis S. D., Baliga B. S. et al. (1972) *J. Biol. Chem.* 247, 3592.

Young V. R., Haverberg L. N., Bilmazes C. et al. (1973) *Metabolism* 22, 1429.

Young V. R. and Munro H. N. (1978) *Fed. Proc.* 37, 2291.

Young V. R., Uauy R., Winterer J. C. et al. (1976a) In: Rockstein M. and Sussman M. L. (ed.), *Nutrition Longevity, Aging.* New York, Academic, pp. 67–102.

Young V. R., Winterer J. C. Munro H. N. et al. (1976b) In: Elias M. F., Eleftheriou B. E. and Elias P. K. (ed.), *Special Review of Experimental Aging Research.* Bar Harbor, Maine, EAR, Inc. pp. 217–252.

3. VITAMINS
A. N. Exton-Smith

Vitamin deficiencies are now rare in younger age groups of the population but for reasons given in Chapter 7 they are more common in old age and assume greater clinical importance. Both low dietary intakes and physical disease — which may interfere with the intake, absorption, metabolism and utilization of vitamins — are responsible. In the case of some vitamins, for example ascorbic acid, dietary lack alone is usually the cause of clinical manifestations, but for the majority of deficiencies dietary lack and endogenous factors act in combination. Only endogenous factors due mainly to disorders of the liver and biliary system produce manifestations of vitamin K deficiency. The most important clinical deficiencies in old age concern vitamins of the B group — folic acid, vitamin B_{12}, — ascorbic acid, vitamin D and vitamin K. Symptoms and signs of deficiencies of vitamins A and E are extremely rare in the elderly.

VITAMIN B COMPLEX DEFICIENCY
Clinical Manifestations
The changes in the mucous membranes of the tongue and lips include:

Cheilosis — red, denuded, often scaly, epithelium at the line of closure of the lips;

Angular stomatitis — greyish white, sodden and swollen epithelium, progressing to fissuring, radiating outwards from the corners of the mouth;

Nasolabial seborrhoea — enlarged follicles around the sides of the nose, and plugged with sebaceous material;

Glossitis — bare, red, smooth tongue with loss of filiform papillae, sometimes associated with fissuring and enlargement of the fungiform papillae.

A high incidence of these changes, which have been attributed to deficiency of riboflavin, nicotinamide and possibly pyridoxine, have been reported by some authors (Brocklehurst et al., 1968; Taylor, 1968).

The most important neurological disturbances are peripheral neuropathy and Wernicke's encephalopathy. They are due principally to deficiency of thiamine, although deficiencies of other B group vitamins (pyridoxine, nicotinic acid and pantothenic acid) may contribute to peripheral neuropathy. Wernicke's encephalopathy is almost certainly due to thiamine deficiency; the clinical features include diplopia and nystagmus, progressing to ophthalmoplegia, and the mental changes of Korsakoff's psychosis – loss of memory, disorientation, confabulation and hallucinations. In Great Britain and the USA it is usually associated with alcoholism, and less often with gastrointestinal disorders causing persistent vomiting. Philip and Smith (1973) have described Wernicke's encephalopathy in old people with accidental hypothermia, and it is likely that the haemorrhagic lesions in the region of the hypothalamus are responsible for the disturbances of temperature regulation. The mental symptoms in Korsakoff's psychosis often improve dramatically when large doses of thiamine, usually with other vitamins of the B group, are given intravenously. Acute confusional states associated with toxic-infective processes, which account for one-third of cases of mental disorder in old people admitted to hospital (Hodkinson, 1973) may in some instances also be attributable to a relative thiamine deficiency. In these patients blood pyruvate levels are often elevated and fall again when the underlying process (e.g., pneumonia) responds to appropriate treatment. These observations need to be confirmed by serial red cell transketolase estimations and it is possible that the development of the acute confusional state is related to the initial status of thiamine nutrition.

The early mental symptoms of nicotinic acid deficiency are irritability, sleeplessness, loss of memory and headaches; later the clinical manifestations of pellagra appear – dermatitis, diarrhoea and dementia. Acute nicotinic acid deficiency, which is found mainly in alcoholics and other malnourished individuals, produces Jolliffe's syndrome – an acute encephalopathy characterized by clouding of consciousness and extrapyramidal rigidity (Jolliffe et al., 1940). As in the case of thiamine deficiency the syndrome is often precipitated by an acute intercurrent infection.

Cardiac manifestations (enlargement of the heart and cardiac failure) occur only in severe degrees of thiamine deficiency. They should be suspected in malnourished old people when cardiac failure occurs without cardiac murmurs and in the absence of other causes.

B Complex Nutritional Status

There is conflict of opinion on the extent to which the tongue mucous membrane lesions reputed to be due to vitamin deficiency can be corrected by vitamin supplementation. Brocklehurst and his colleagues (1968) concluded from a controlled trial in 80 elderly in-patients that there is chronic vitamin deficiency in a large number of elderly people which can be reversed by large doses of vitamin supplements for long periods. Later Dymock and Brocklehurst (1973) repeated their earlier studies and used single vitamin supplementation on 77 old people in hospital who survived for one year's clinical trial. Riboflavin therapy was associated with significant improvement in cheilosis, and possibly in angular stomatitis; and nicotinamide produced a significant improvement in the dorsum of the tongue. On the other hand, MacLeod (1972) and Berry and Darke (1972) failed to confirm these findings. The latter investigators found a fungal infection in 90 per cent of the subjects who had changes in the dorsal surface of the tongue and they considered that this was the most likely cause of the changes.

In the Nutrition Survey of the Elderly (DHSS, 1972) a special attempt was made to relate changes in the mucous membranes to riboflavin deficiency. Of the 778 subjects examined 57 were diagnosed as having either angular stomatitis or cheilosis. There was no statistical difference in the mean riboflavin intakes in those with lip lesions compared with those without these lesions. Out of the 23 subjects who had very low intakes of riboflavin (less than 0·7 mg for males and 0·55 mg for females) 4 subjects had lip lesions. It was concluded that although there may be some element of clinical ariboflavinosis in the elderly population the number must be very small and in general the riboflavin status appeared to be satisfactory.

Significance of Deficiencies

Brin (1964, 1968) has investigated the biochemical changes in thiamine deficiency. Thiamine adequacy was assessed by determining its urinary excretion level, by measurement of the erythrocyte transketolase (TK) activity and by calculation of the TPP effect. In the last test thiamine pyrophosphate (TPP), the co-enzyme of thiamine, is added to the haemo-lysed cells and the TPP effect is calculated from the increment of TK activity due to the addition of TPP and by then expressing this as a per-centage of the TK activity of unenriched blood. After 5 days on a thiamine-depleted diet urinary thiamine excretion is reduced to 50 μg daily; after about 10 days the TK activity is depressed with a positive TPP effect of about 15 per cent and the urinary thiamine is reduced to 25 μg; the third or 'physiological' stage is reached by 21 days when the urinary thiamine is 0–25 μg daily and the TK activity is reduced 15–25 per cent with a TPP effect up to 30 per cent. By the time clinical manifestations of deficiency appeared the TK activity was reduced more than 35 per cent and the TPP effect was in excess of 40 per cent. It was noted that the urinary thiamine excretion reached a minimum level in 12 days and once this level was reached it was not possible to differentiate between a pre-clinical deficiency state and severe disease by this measure alone. Values of TPP effect below 15 per cent were taken as normal; above this critical level there was found to be a definitive curve of relationship between TK activity and TPP effect.

In a study of 233 subjects aged 44–94 years Brin (1968) found thia-mine deficiency in 37 per cent as judged by reduced thiamine excretion and in 5 per cent if based on a TPP effect of greater than 15 per cent. In a study of 80 elderly long-stay patients Griffiths (1968) found that only 21 were not thiamine deficient based on a less strict criterion of a TPP effect of more than 10 per cent. The subjects were re-examined at 3, 6, 9 and 12 months after thiamine supplementation and only one failed to return to the normal level after one year.

The riboflavin status of 128 old people has been investigated by Thurnham (1972) in a study of accidental hypothermia based on a random sample of the elderly population in the London Borough of Camden. The erythrocyte glutathione reductase activity (EGR) and the percentage stimulation of EGR by flavin adenine dinucleotide (FAD) were measured. A percent stimulation of greater than 30 per cent (usually regarded as the upper limit of normal) was found in 18 per cent of the men and in 19 per cent of the women. Thus it is considered that there may be marginal riboflavin deficiency in about one-fifth of the elderly population. Although the true significance of this marginal deficiency is at present unknown these laboratory tests serve to identify those individuals who might benefit from vitamin supplementation to prevent the appearance of acute deficiency disease.

FOLATE DEFICIENCY
Clinical Manifestations
The main clinical findings are anaemia and changes in the nervous system and mucous membrane of the tongue. The anaemia is megaloblastic, characterized by abnormal nucleated red cell precursors (megaloblasts) in the bone marrow and macrocytes in the peripheral blood. There is associated leucopenia with hypersegmentation of the neutrophils, and the number of platelets may be reduced. There may be the complaint of soreness or burning of the tongue, and the surface may be red due to acute glossitis; but it is more commonly smooth, shiny and atrophic. In patients with chronic neurological diseases, especially peripheral neuropathy, the changes including megaloblastic anaemia are more often due to folate deficiency than to vitamin B_{12} deficiency (Grant et al., 1965). Mental changes may precede the anaemia; they are non-specific and include mild confusion, depression, apathy and intellectual impairment. Cases of dementia due to folate deficiency have been reported and Strachan and Henderson (1965) noted a response in 2 patients with dementia to prolonged folate administration.

Causes
The main causes of folate deficiency in the elderly are inadequate intake, malabsorption, increased utilization and impaired effectiveness. In contrast to vitamin B_{12} deficiency, dietary inadequacy of folate is an important cause of deficiency. A mixed diet contains 500–800 µg folate per day; but as it is mainly in the reduced form, the folate is readily destroyed by sunlight, oxidation and cooking. The minimum requirements are 50–100 µg per day, but many times this amount may be required if there is increased utilization. Dietary deficiency is often associated with mental and physical disorders interfering with shopping and cooking, as well as

with poverty. Absorption of folate occurs in the upper small intestine and it may be impaired in gluten enteropathy and in other conditions giving rise to malabsorption syndrome. Folate requirements increase when cell turnover increases, e.g. in haemolytic anaemia, myeloproliferative syndromes, carcinoma, myeloma and in certain chronic inflammatory diseases such as tuberculosis and Crohn's disease. Under certain conditions the effectiveness of available folate is impaired – vitamin C deficiency inhibits folate co-enzymes and in scurvy impaired folate metabolism can lead to megaloblastic anaemia (see p. 32). Barbiturates and anticonvulsants interfere with folate metabolism and are responsible for manifestations of folate deficiency in epileptic patients.

Folate Status
Although a folate-free diet quickly leads to lowering of serum folate levels, many months elapse before clinical or haematological changes develop. In a survey of elderly patients admitted to a geriatric department in a South London hospital, Hurdle and Williams (1966) found low serum folate levels (less than 5 ng/ml) in one-third of the patients. A deficiency of body stores was indicated by a positive FIGLU test in 50 per cent of the patients with folate deficiency. A nutritional origin was suggested by the finding of an increase in the incidence with greater severity of disability; two-thirds of those unable to look after themselves were folate deficient. Read et al. (1965) in Bristol found that 80 per cent of entrants to old people's homes had folate deficiency, based on a serum folate level of less than 6 ng/ml. Such a lower limit, however, does not represent a very strict criterion of deficiency. In the Nutritional Survey of the Elderly (DHSS, 1972) serum folate levels of less than 3 ng/ml were found in 14·6 per cent of the subjects living at home. Red cell folate levels of less than 150 ng/ml were found in 16·1 per cent indicating chronic folate deficiency; more severe degrees of deficiency with red cell folate concentrations of less than 100 ng/ml were found in 3·7 per cent of the subjects studied. There was a significant correlation between serum and red cell folate concentrations ($P<0·01$). Batata et al. (1967) in Oxford found that 10 per cent of patients over the age of 60 had serum folate levels of less than 2·1 ng/ml. A nutritional origin was suspected since the more severe the disability (and in consequence the greater the inability of the patient to look after himself) the more likely was there to be folate deficiency; there was found to be a statistically significant relationship between organic brain disease and low folate levels. Sneath et al. (1973) examined the relationship between folate status and dementia in patients admitted to the geriatric department. In a series of 115 consecutive admissions 14 patients were diagnosed as having dementia. Their mean red cell folate concentration (279 ng/ml) was significantly lower than the mean (394 ng/ml) for the group as a whole and also significantly lower than that in 8 patients with carcinoma, 14 patients with congestive cardiac failure and 23 patients with hemiplegia.

There was also some correlation between intellectual function as assessed on a 16 point mental test score and the red cell folate concentration in those with low red cell folate levels (below 200 ng/ml). Thus the association between poor folate nutrition and dementia was confirmed in this study. It was thought that the dementia leads to inadequate dietary intake and in turn to folate deficiency, but the possibility that folate deficiency itself leads to impaired mental function could not be excluded.

VITAMIN B_{12} DEFICIENCY
Clinical Manifestations
The clinical features of vitamin B_{12} deficiency include megaloblastic anaemia, glossitis, subacute combined degeneration of the cord, peripheral neuropathy and mental changes. The onset of symptoms is usually insidious so that the anaemia may be severe when the patient first presents. The apathy, tiredness, weakness and breathlessness due to the anaemia are difficult to evaluate in the elderly patient. The skin may have a yellow tinge. Although the classic raw 'red-beef' tongue can occur, the tongue surface is more often smooth, pale and atrophic. Paraesthesiae in the hands and feet, unsteadiness on standing and weakness of the legs occur in patients with peripheral neuropathy and pyramidal and posterior column lesions. Mental changes may predominate; some may be due specifically to vitamin B_{12} deficiency since it is known that the cortical degeneration occurring in B_{12} deficiency is similar to that which occurs in the spinal cord. Shulman (1972) found a higher incidence of psychiatric symptoms in patients with anaemia due to B_{12} deficiency than in those patients whose anaemia was due to other causes. He considers that psychiatrists should be aware of the possibility of B_{12} deficiency in patients with anaemia or after gastrectomy or where fatigue, mental confusion or dementia are of unknown origin.

Causes
Vitamin B_{12} occurs in most animal tissues but not in plants. It is absorbed in the ileum after binding with intrinsic factor (IF), a mucoprotein secreted by the gastric parietal cells. Apart from vegans, in whom dietary deficiency of vitamin B_{12} may occur, the deficiency is due to malabsorption. This may be the result of gastric lesions as in pernicious anaemia, chronic atrophic gastritis and after partial or total gastrectomy; or of intestinal lesions in such conditions as gluten-sensitive enteropathy, jejunal diverticulosis, blind-loop syndrome, fistula and after ileal resection. The commonest cause is pernicious anaemia, in which the vitamin B_{12} deficiency is secondary to lack of IF secretion. The gastric lesion is believed to be an autoimmune phenomenon, since antibodies to both IF and parietal cells are found in the gastric juice of patients with pernicious anaemia.

Vitamin B_{12} Status

Pernicious anaemia is a disease of later life occurring more frequently as age advances. The overall prevalence in the UK is $0.1-0.2$ per cent, but over the age of 60 it is about 1 per cent. MacLennan et al. (1973) found an incidence of 2.5 per cent in two surveys of people age 65 and over living at home in Glasgow and Kilsyth. The incidence of pernicious anaemia is higher in Scotland than in England, and it is higher in the North of England than in the South. In the general population the incidence of achlorhydria, chronic gastritis and circulating antibodies to parietal cells rises steadily after middle age. These changes could account for the progressive fall in serum vitamin B_{12} levels with advancing age which have been reported (Cape and Shinton, 1961). It is believed, however, that the serum levels of vitamin B_{12} may also be affected by the tissue status of other haemopoietic nutrients, notably iron and folate. Thus low B_{12} levels accompany iron deficiency and they rise following the administration of oral iron. Similarly, low serum B_{12} levels are found in about one-third of patients with nutritional megaloblastic anaemia due to folate deficiency, and treatment with folic acid alone restores the serum B_{12} level (Mollin et al., 1962). It can be concluded that vitamin B_{12} status cannot always be accurately assessed by measurement of serum levels.

ASCORBIC ACID DEFICIENCY

Clinical Features

Scurvy is still occasionally seen in the elderly, especially in men, and the manifestations include swelling and bleeding from the gums (not seen in edentulous individuals), weakness, anaemia, extensive haemorrhages in the skin of the legs and arms ('sheet' haemorrhages) and sometimes haemorrhages at other sites. Mental changes, especially apathy and depression, are often present in vitamin C deficiency (Walker, 1968).

Anaemia is common in scurvy; it is usually normocytic or macrocytic with normoblastic or macronormoblastic erythropoiesis, but cases of true megaloblastic anaemia have been reported (Goldberg, 1963; Hyams and Ross, 1963). The origin of anaemia is often multifactorial: haemolysis, bleeding, dietary deficiency of iron and derangement of red cell metabolism have been incriminated (Cox, 1968). Megaloblastic change has been attributed either to an associated dietary folate deficiency or to impairment of folate metabolism in scurvy. Stokes et al. (1975) have shown that megaloblastic anaemia of scurvy is caused in part by removal of tetrahydrofolates from the metabolic pool due to oxidation to 10-formyl folic acid. It is believed that an important role of ascorbic acid in metabolism is to prevent the oxidation of the tetrahydrofolates and thus to maintain the availability of the folate metabolic pool. Russell et al. (1968) have shown that vitamin C deficiency may play a part in maintaining gastrointestinal haemorrhage which had been precipitated initially by gastric irritants such as aspirin.

It has been known for some time that wound healing may be delayed in vitamin C deficiency and the administration of vitamin C may promote the healing of pressure sores by increasing collagen formation (Burr and Rajan, 1972).

Vitamin C Status

Although overt manifestations of deficiency are rare, the body stores of vitamin C in many old people are diminished. Low levels of leucocyte ascorbic acid (LAA) have been reported by several observers: the levels are lower in the elderly than in younger subjects (Bowers and Kubik, 1965; Andrews et al., 1969); lower in winter than in summer (Andrews et al., 1966); lower in men than in women (Milne et al., 1971); and smokers have lower LAA levels compared with non-smokers (Brook and Grimshaw, 1968). Furthermore, diminished ascorbic acid levels have been reported in institutionalized old people (Kataria et al., 1965; Andrews and Brook, 1966). They have been attributed to the effects of cooking in institutions of such foods as potatoes; the delay in delivery of the meal to the recipient; and to an inadequate supply of fruit and fruit juices (Andrews, 1973). Similar factors may be responsible for the inferior vitamin C status of old people receiving meals-on-wheels, mainly the housebound. These meals are cooked in institutions and are kept hot for several hours in containers before they are delivered. Stanton (1971) has shown that 90 per cent of the vitamin C may be destroyed before the meal is served. Davies et al. (1973), in a study of a meals-on-wheels service supplied on average two to three days per week, have demonstrated that the vitamin C intake may be considerably less on those days on which the old person receives a domiciliary meal compared with days on which he or she does the cooking at home. The low levels of LAA in certain old people are not a natural accompaniment of ageing since by feeding with ascorbic acid they can be brought to levels seen in younger people (Andrews et al., 1966).

In a study in Edinburgh, Milne and his colleagues (1971) found that LAA levels were significantly higher in July to December compared with those from whom blood samples were taken during the rest of the year. Slightly more than half the subjects had intakes of less than 30 mg per day and a significantly greater proportion had low intakes in the months October to March compared with the months April to September. Vitamin C intake was correlated with LAA level and it was found that LAA levels increased in parallel with, but lagged behind, seasonal increases in vitamin C intakes. Similar findings were reported in the Nutrition Survey of the Elderly (DHSS, 1972) and there was a correlation between LAA levels and vitamin C intake (Darke, 1972).

Significance of Low Tissue Stores

The Edinburgh study and other dietary surveys disclose that there is a significant number of old people whose intake of vitamin C is less than

10 mg/d, which is known to be the amount required to prevent or cure scurvy (Bartley et al., 1953). The recommended allowance of 30 mg daily (DHSS, 1969) takes into account the considerable individual variations in requirements and increased requirements due to stress. Although a high proportion of the elderly population consumes less than 30 mg per day the majority will not suffer any ill-effects. Our assessment of vitamin C requirements is handicapped by lack of knowledge of the tissue levels needed for health. Windsor and Williams (1970) by measuring total hydroxyproline excretion (THP) in response to vitamin C, found that THP increased when the initial LAA content was less than 15 μg/10^8 w.b.c., but when the LAA level was higher than this the response to vitamin C supplementation failed to occur. A level of LAA less than 15 μg/10^8 w.b.c. is usually taken to indicate biochemical deficiency. In very old people there may be considerable individual variability. The scatter diagrams for LAA and average daily vitamin C intake based on data from the DHSS Nutrition Survey of the Elderly (Darke, 1972) show that there are some subjects, especially the men, who have high vitamin C intakes (>50 mg/d) yet have low LAA levels of less than 15 μg/10^8 w.b.c.

Wilson et al. (1972) have studied the relationship between LAA levels and mortality in aged hospital patients. The mortality was found to be 47 per cent within 4 weeks of admission for those whose initial LAA levels were less than 12 μg/10^8 w.b.c. compared with 10 per cent when the LAA was greater than 25 μg/10^8 ($P<0.01$). Subsequent investigation, however, showed that mortality was not directly related to LAA levels but to the severity of the illness which in turn, influenced the tissue stores of vitamin C (Wilson et al., 1973). In the follow-up study administration of vitamin C failed to produce an increase in LAA levels in many of the subjects; nor did it influence mortality. Thus it is believed that many illnesses occurring in elderly patients depress LAA concentration; moreover, a number of drugs used in clinical practice, for example, tetracycline (Windsor et al., 1972) also depress LAA levels.

VITAMIN D DEFICIENCY AND OSTEOMALACIA
Vitamin D deficiency produces osteomalacia, a generalized disease of bone characterized by a deficient calcification of a normal bone matrix. Histological examination reveals an increase in the amount of osteoid, that is, non-calcified matrix around the bone trabeculae.

Clinical Manifestations
In the early stages the patient often complains of vague pains in a variety of sites and these are usually dismissed as 'rheumatism'. Later the pain becomes more persistent and localized to the bones which are extremely tender to pressure. The patient becomes shorter owing to deformities of the trunk — usually kyphosis — and on radiography the intervertebral discs are often ballooned and the soft vertebral bodies become biconcave

('cod-fish vertebrae'). Other bones may become deformed such as the sternum, the pelvis and the femoral necks. Another characteristic finding on radiographic examination is the appearance of Looser's zones or pseudo-fractures. These are bands of decalcification perpendicular or oblique to the surface of the bone and on either side of the translucency there may be a denser band of callus. They occur in only about one-third of cases of osteomalacia, but as they are pathognomonic of osteomalacia a skeletal survey should be conducted in suspected cases, particular attention being paid to the pubic rami, the femoral neck, the ribs, the border of the scapula, the upper end of the humerus and less frequently the shafts of the tibia, fibula, radius and ulna. In addition to Looser's zones true spontaneous fractures occur.

Muscular weakness is often striking. For many years this has been regarded as a typical feature of rickets, but only recently has it been recognized in osteomalacia. It usually takes the form of a proximal myopathy affecting the muscles of the pelvic and shoulder girdles. The patient may complain of difficulty in climbing stairs and in getting up from a chair; when walking the patient may have a typical 'waddling gait'. When the shoulder girdle muscles are involved the patient is unable to raise the arms and perform such activities as brushing the hair.

Aetiology

The vitamin D deficiency leading to osteomalacia in old people is often multifactorial in origin. It has been attributed to a fall in dietary intake of vitamin D (Exton-Smith et al., 1966); a reduction in exposure to sunlight (Stamp and Round, 1974); malabsorption, including gluten enteropathy (Moss et al., 1965); gastrectomy (Clark et al., 1964); increased physiological requirement for vitamin D (Dent, 1970); and impaired conversion of 25-hydroxycholecalciferol to the active 1,25-dihydroxycholecalciferol due to a decline in renal function in old age (Fraser and Kodicek, 1970; Lund et al., 1975). The many conditions which may give rise to vitamin D deficiency in old age account for the fact that osteomalacia is more common in the elderly than in younger age groups.

Vitamin D Status

The state of vitamin D nutrition of two groups of elderly women has been assessed by Smith et al. (1964). For women living in Michigan (average age 60·6 years) the level of vitamin D in the blood as determined by the serum antirachitic activity was significantly lower in those subjects with low bone density compared with those having normal bones, and the level showed marked seasonal variation. By contrast for a group of women of similar age living in Puerto Rico, where there is much greater exposure to sunlight and higher vitamin D content of food, the incidence of skeletal rarefaction was much lower, the serum vitamin D levels were much higher, and there was no seasonal variation. Using the more precise index of radio-stereo-assay of 25-hydroxycholecalciferol levels, Stamp and Round (1974) have shown similar seasonal variations in both young and old subjects. They conclude that summer sunlight is an important, and possibly the chief, determinant of vitamin D nutrition in Britain. In this study, the older people who participated in a nutrition survey in the London Borough of Camden had significantly lower levels of 25-hydroxycholecalciferol than those found in the younger subjects. In this respect, housebound old people (Exton-Smith et al., 1972) may be at the greatest disadvantage since they lack exposure to sunlight and often have very low dietary intakes; 48 per cent of housebound women aged 70–79 years had a dietary intake of less than 30 iu per day compared with 13 per cent of active women of similar age.

The question has recently arisen whether vitamin D deficiency is of clinical importance in the absence of the usual features of osteomalacia. Examination of iliac crest biopsy material shows that 20–40 per cent of patients with fracture of the proximal femur have histological evidence of osteomalacia (Aaron et al., 1974a and b; Faccini et al., 1976). There is also the possibility that long-continued mild vitamin D deficiency of insufficient severity to cause osteomalacia may lead to accelerated bone loss and thus contribute to the pathogenesis of osteoporosis. These problems are discussed in Chapter 11.

There is obvious need for improvement of the vitamin D status in a considerable number of elderly people. This could be achieved by dietary supplementation or by exposure to ultraviolet light. Irrespective of whether vitamin D deficiency is concerned in the pathogenesis of osteoporosis these measures might be expected to reduce the fracture rate, particularly in those individuals whose disabilities confine them to home or an institution.

VITAMIN K DEFICIENCY

The dietary sources of vitamin K occur as either phylloquinone (vitamin K_1) in vegetable oils and leafy plants, or as menoquinones (vitamin K_2) which are produced by many varieties of bacteria. Vitamin K is synthesized in the colon by the normal gut flora. The naturally occurring phylloquinone and menoquinones are absorbed adequately from the small intestine only in the presence of bile salts. They are stored in small amounts in the liver where they are required for the synthesis of four separate coagulation factors – prothrombin, and factors VII, IX and X. Coumarin-type drugs (e.g. warfarin, phenindione) inhibit the action of vitamin K in the synthesis of these coagulation factors.

The most important causes of vitamin K deficiency are obstructive jaundice, causing impaired absorption of vitamin K_1 and K_2, and hepatocellular damage, in which there is impaired synthesis of the coagulation factors. On rare occasions deficiency may develop in malnourished old people who are given a broad-spectrum antibiotic which interferes with the bacterial synthesis of vitamin K in the gut. Biliary obstruction quickly leads to a decline in the hepatic stores of vitamin K and hypoprothrombinaemia appears within a few weeks.

The clinical manifestations are severe subcutaneous haemorrhages and bleeding from other sites.

The vitamin K deficiency in biliary obstruction can be rapidly corrected by administration of vitamin K parenterally. When, however, the cause of the deficiency is hepatocellular damage the response to vitamin K may be poor, since the liver's ability to synthesize prothrombin and the other three coagulation factors is impaired.

REFERENCES

Aaron J. E., Gallagher J. C., Anderson J. et al. (1974a) *Lancet* 1, 229.
Aaron J. E., Gallagher J. C. and Nordin B. E. C. (1974b) *Lancet* 2, 84.
Andrews J. (1973) *Gerontol. Clin. (Basel)* 15, 221.
Andrews J. and Brook M. (1966) *Lancet* 1, 1350.
Andrews J., Brook M. and Allen M. A. A. (1966) *Gerontol. Clin. (Basel)* 8, 257.
Andrews J., Letcher M. and Brook M. (1969) *Br. Med. J.* 2, 416.
Bartley W., Krebs H. A. and O'Brien J. R. P. (1953) *Vitamin C Requirements of Human Adults, MRC Special Report Series No. 280.* London, HMSO.
Batata M., Spray G. H., Bolton F. G. et al. (1967) *Br. Med. J.* 2, 667.
Berry W. T. C. and Darke S. (1972) *Age Ageing* 1, 177.
Bowers E. F. and Kubik M. M. (1965) *Br. J. Clin. Pract.* 19, 147.
Brin M. (1964) *J. Am. Med. Assoc.* 187, 762.
Brin M. (1968) In: Exton-Smith A. N. and Scott D. L. (*see* General References).
Brocklehurst J., Griffiths L. L., Taylor G. F. et al. (1968) *Gerontol. Clin. (Basel)* 10, 309.
Brook J. and Grimshaw J. J. (1968) *Am. J. Clin. Nutr.* 21, 1254.
Burr R. G. and Rajan K. T. (1972) *Br. J. Nutr.* 28, 275.
Cape R. D. T. and Shinton N. K. (1961) *Gerontol. Clin. (Basel)* 3, 23.
Clark C. G., Crooks J., Dawson A. A. et al. (1964) *Lancet* 1, 734.
Cox E. V. (1968) *Vitam. Horm.* 26, 635.
Darke S. (1972) Requirements for Vitamins in Old Age, In: Carlson L. A. (ed.), *Nutrition in Old Age.* Uppsala, Almquist & Wiksell.
Davies L., Hastrop K. and Bender A. E. (1973) *Mod. Geriat.* 3, 290.
Dent C. E. (1970) *Proc. R. Soc. Med.* 63, 401.
DHSS (1969) 120 (*see* General References).
DHSS (1972) 3 (*see* General References).
Dymock S. M. and Brocklehurst J. C. (1973) *Age Ageing* 2, 172.
Exton-Smith A. N., Hodkinson H. M. and Stanton B. R. (1966) *Lancet* 1, 999.
Exton-Smith A. N., Stanton B. R. and Windsor A. C. M. (1972) (*see* General References).
Faccini J. M., Exton-Smith A. N. and Boyde A. (1976) *Lancet* 1, 1089.
Fraser D. R. and Kodicek E. (1970) *Nature* 228, 764.
Goldberg A. (1963) *Q. J. Med.* 32, 51.
Grant H. C., Hoffbrand A. V. and Wells D. G. (1965) *Lancet* 2, 763.
Griffiths L. L. (1968) In: Exton-Smith A. N. and Scott D. L. (*see* General References).
Hodkinson H. M. (1973) *J. R. Coll. Physicians Lond.* 7, 305.
Hurdle A. D. F. and Williams T. C. P. (1966) *Br. Med. J.* 2, 202.
Hyams D. E. and Ross E. J. (1963) *Br. J. Clin. Pract.* 17, 332.
Jolliffe N., Bowman K. M., Rosenblum L. A. et al. (1940) *J. Am. Med. Assoc.* 114, 307.

Kataria M. S., Rao D. B. and Curtis R. C. (1965) *Gerontol. Clin. (Basel)* 7, 189.
Lund B., Hjorth I., Kjaer I. et al. (1975) *Lancet* 2, 1168.
MacLennan W. J., Andrews G. R., MacLeod C. et al. (1973) *Q. J. Med.* 42, 1.
MacLeod R. D. M. (1972) *Age Ageing* 1, 99.
Milne J. S., Lonergan M. E., Williamson J. et al. (1971) *Br. Med. J.* 4, 383.
Mollin D. L., Waters A. H. and Harriss E. (1962) In: Heinrich H. C. (ed.), *Vitamin B and Intrinsic Factor*, Vol. 2. Stuttgart, Enke.
Moss A. J., Waterhouse C. and Terry R. (1965) *New Engl. J. Med.* 272, 825.
Philip G. and Smith J. F. (1973) *Lancet* 2, 122.
Read A. E., Gough K. R., Pardoe J. L. et al. (1965) *Br. Med. J.* 2, 843.
Russell R. I., Williamson J. M., Goldberg A. et al. (1968) *Lancet* 2, 603.
Shulman R. (1972) *Can. Psychiatr. Assoc. J.* 17, 205.
Smith R. W., Rizek J., Frame B. et al. (1964) *Am. J. Nutr.* 14, 98.
Sneath P., Chanarin I., Hodkinson H. M. et al. (1973) *Age Ageing* 2, 177.
Stamp T. C. B. and Round J. M. (1974) *Nature* 247, 563.
Stanton B. R. (1971) *Meals for the Elderly*. London, King Edward's Hospital Fund.
Stokes P. L., Melikian V., Leeming R. L. et al. (1975) *Am. J. Clin. Nutr.* 28, 126.
Strachan R. W. and Henderson J. G. (1965) *Q. J. Med.* 34, 303.
Taylor G. F. (1968) In: Exton-Smith A. N. and Scott D. L. (*see* General References).
Thurnham D. (1972) Personal communication.
Walker A. (1968) *Br. J. Dermatol.* 80, 625.
Wilson T. S., Datta S. B., Murrell J. S. et al. (1973) *Age Ageing* 2, 163.
Wilson T. S., Weeks M. M., Mukherjee S. K. et al. (1972) *Gerontol. Clin. (Basel)* 14, 17.
Windsor A. C. M., Hobbs C. B., Treby D. A. et al. (1972) *Br. Med. J.* 1, 214.
Windsor A. C. M. and Williams C. B. (1970) *Br. Med. J.* 1, 732.

4. POTASSIUM AND MAGNESIUM
T. G. Judge

POTASSIUM

Potassium is the main intracellular cation. It is responsible for the cell membrane action potential and as a result is essential for the function of the sodium pump, for some aspects of nerve conduction and for part of the regulation of muscle irritability.

Total body potassium in middle life is some 3000 mmol, but in old age this falls to some 2500 mmol (MacLennan et al., 1977). Part of this reduction must be related to increased body water and reduced non-fat body mass which occurs with ageing, but part appears to be an absolute reduction. Further reduction in total body potassium occurs in cardiac failure (Cox et al., 1971) and following the use of diuretics (Ibrahim et al., 1978). Large changes in total body potassium occur without significant change in the serum potassium level. This is not surprising since only 2 per cent of total body potassium is in the extracellular compartment. Conversely, change in serum potassium outside the normal confidence limits is of considerable clinical significance. In one series, based on study of 1000 consecutive admissions to hospital, it was found that 1 old person in 10 had a pathologically low serum potassium on admission (Judge, 1968). When allowance is made for dehydration and haemoconcentration the incidence of significant hypokalaemia is greater.

As a result of the fundamental role of the ion in human physiology, a wide range of symptoms results both from depletion and from excess. Many of the anomalies in clinical practice which arise in connection with potassium metabolism can be explained when it is understood that the intracellular/extracellular ratio is of greater importance in most instances than absolute levels.

Potassium depletion can result in muscle weakness, apathy, confusion, constipation (Judge, 1968) abdominal distension, paralytic ileus, cardiac arrhythmias (Pick, 1966) reduced cardiac output with resultant cardiac failure and hence oedema (Allison et al., 1972), impaired renal concentration and thus polyuria and thirst, increased liability to unwanted drug effects (from digoxin for example) and sudden death, particularly when acute depletion results from sudden migration of the ion during the treatment of severe anaemia (Lawson et al., 1972) or of diabetic coma (Alberti et al., 1973).

The classically described ECG changes of potassium depletion, reduction in the size of the T wave and ST depression, are an extremely variable feature. Reduction of hand-grip strength has been described by Cowan and Judge (1969) in a paired series where correction had been made for predicted change due to age and sex difference. Burr et al. (1975) failed to confirm these findings and found only age and sex differences.

Normal serum values for potassium in later life for healthy people do not differ significantly from the reference ranges given by most laboratories. The 95 per cent confidence limit is usually taken as 3·8—5·4 mmol. Leask et al. (1973) found 4·4 ± 0·4 mmol/l to be the central value in a normal population of old people in the community in a random sample. Blood levels outside this range are almost always the result of disease and worthy of treatment.

The source of body potassium is the diet, which in middle life often contains 50—150 mmol per day (Davidson et al., 1973). In the elderly, this intake is often much less (Judge and MacLeod, 1968; Davies, 1973; MacLeod et al. 1975). As a direct result of poor intake, many old people are at risk of developing depletion. Because of varying absorption, varying utilization and varying loss in different individuals, the daily requirement of potassium is uncertain: the figure of 60 mmol per day is probably generous, but 60 per cent of women and 40 per cent of men failed to reach this intake in one sample of the population (Judge and MacLeod, 1968); later work (MacLeod et al., 1975) confirmed this finding. In the latter random population sample 9 per cent of men and 14 per cent of women took less than 40 mmol of potassium per day.

Many foods are rich in potassium — for example, citrus fruits, meat and fish — but the elderly often have rigid food habits. MacLeod et al. (1975) showed that the main dietary sources were as follows: milk (which accounted for 19 per cent of the mean intake), potatoes (16 per cent), meat and meat dishes (14 per cent), beverages (10 per cent) biscuits and cakes (8 per cent) and bread (6 per cent). It has been shown by Dall et al. (1971) that young hospital in-patients offered the same choice of food as elderly in-patients select a diet with an adequate potassium content, whereas the older patients select a diet deficient in this mineral. There is no doubt that a diet containing less than 30 mmol of potassium per day leads inevitably to potassium depletion as measured by an abnormally low serum level (Kaul et al., 1965) — the most significant and serious measure: and it is likely that intakes between 30 and 60 mmol/d will cause problems in some elderly patients.

Potassium is lost from the extracellular space through the intestinal mucosa; through the kidney (either as a result of glomerular filtration or as a result of impaired tubular reabsorption), or through the cell membrane of any body cell (Zilva and Pannall, 1975). Urinary loss is related to intake but in contrast to losses in younger people, irreducible minimal loss in the elderly may be as high as 20 mmol/d (Judge et al., 1974). Increased intestinal loss occurs in vomiting and diarrhoea; in the presence of alimentary fistulae; from mucus-secreting tumours of the rectum; from mucus loss in the pseudo-diarrhoea of faecal impaction; and ureteric transplants into the colon (Whitby et al., 1977).

Reduced renal tubular reabsorption occurs most commonly as a result of diuretic therapy, but is also found in sodium retention syndromes, hyperaldosteronism, Cushing's syndrome, overdosage of corticosteroids, use of carbenoxolone, acidosis, hyperchloraemia and in potassium-losing nephropathies (Zilva and Pannall, 1975). A low serum potassium has also been reported in influenza (Crocket, 1970) and in recent stroke, purgation, chronic urinary infection, anorexia and following the use of reserpine and chlorpromazine (Judge, 1968).

Retention of potassium occurs following the use of potassium-sparing diuretics such as triamterene (Dyaside; Dytac) and triamterene-containing preparations such as Dytide, and amiloride (Midamor) or amiloride-containing preparations such as Moduretic. These preparations are of great value as potassium-conserving diuretics, but they must *never* be combined with the use of potassium supplements, because a dangerously high level of serum potassium can result. They should be used with care in the elderly because they can cause a rising blood urea. Their use is attractive in reducing the number of tablets to be taken each day, especially since the combined preparations of conventional diuretics with potassium contain too little potassium to be effective.

Retention of potassium may lead to lethargy, confusion and asthenia indistinguishable from the symptoms of potassium depletion. Cardiac arrhythmias may also occur, often bradycardia associated with heart block. Death may result from cardiac arrest (Robson, 1974).

Treatment of potassium depletion is with oral potassium chloride, if the patient is able to swallow and not vomiting. In other circumstances, intravenous potassium chloride is used. When intravenous medication is indicated but unwise because of fear of circulatory overload, or because of lack of medical or nursing resources, subcutaneous therapy may be used. Of the oral preparations of potassium chloride available, those containing the salt in an unmodified form or an enteric-coated form must be avoided because of the risk of small bowel ulceration (Morgenstern et al., 1965). Slow-release preparations of potassium are widely used, as are effervescent tablets. The standard preparations in the UK are: potassium chloride slow tablets BNF (Slow-K, Leo-K, K Contin) and potassium chloride effervescent tablets BNF (Sando-K, Kloref). Preparations of potassium bicarbonate should not be used, since the bicarbonate iron increases the alkalotic hypochloraemia which often coexists with potassium depletion and leads to further loss of potassium (Judge, 1973). It is significant that when potassium bicarbonate was the standard preparation for the treatment of potassium depletion, the death rate of patients with this condition was much higher than it is now when the chloride is used. On occasion, however, potassium chloride fails to correct potassium depletion for reasons which are obscure. In these cases, it is worth a trial of a non-chloride containing supplement such as potassium gluconate (Katorin) (Judge, 1969; 1973).

When potassium chloride is given intravenously, a rate of 20 mmol per hour must not be exceeded because of the danger of cardiac arrhythmia. For subcutaneous use, one ampoule of potassium chloride (BP) which contains 20 mmol is added to 500 ml of normal saline.

The management of potassium excess involves the restriction of dietary intake. Rapid fall in serum potassium level can be achieved by the use of glucose and insulin — 50 g of glucose by mouth followed by 20 units of soluble insulin given subcutaneously (Robson, 1974). Resonium A (an ion-exchange resin) is effective by mouth or as a retention enema in a dose of 30 g in a small amount of water four times a day. Peritoneal dialysis and extracorporeal dialysis are effective when ethical considerations do not preclude their use in this age group.

MAGNESIUM

Magnesium, like potassium, is predominantly an intracellular ion. The total body magnesium in middle life is 1000 mmol, about half of which is in bone. Most of the remainder is found in liver and muscle cells (Davidson et al., 1973). Only a very small amount is found in the extracellular space, and of this some $0 \cdot 75 - 1 \cdot 0$ mmol/l is to be found in the plasma. Although these figures represent the reference range in adult life (Whitby et al., 1977), Leask et al. (1973) found a value of $0 \cdot 8 \pm 0 \cdot 1$ mmol/l in a normal elderly population.

The physiological role of magnesium is to activate intracellular enzymes and to promote glucose metabolism (Gaddum, 1959; Davidson et al., 1973). Depletion is probably more common than is presently recognized, and occurs in roughly the same circumstances as potassium depletion. The source of body magnesium is the diet, which in middle life contains approximately 20 mmol/d (Whitby et al., 1977). One-third of this is absorbed in healthy people, the remainder being lost in the gut. In the elderly, the daily intake ranges from 14 ± 7 mmol in men aged 69—74 to $9 \cdot 5 \pm 3 \cdot 5$ mmol in women aged 75 and over (MacLeod et al., 1975). It is thought that the minimal daily requirement is of the order of 8—12 mmol (Recommended Daily Allowances, 1964). It would appear that 89 per cent of women and 78 per cent of men take in less than $9 \cdot 6$ mmol/d (MacLeod et al., 1975).

Magnesium absorption resembles that of calcium (although vitamin D is not required) and takes place in the small bowel. The amount absorbed depends on the dietary phosphate and calcium level since competition occurs (Whitby et al., 1977) and is also related to the amount of phytic acid in the diet. The current enthusiasm for high-fibre diets which contain a large amount of phytin increases the risk of magnesium (and calcium) depletion. Although chlorophyll contains magnesium and is widely distributed in nature, the principal sources of this substance in the diet of the elderly are bread, milk, breakfast cereals, biscuits and cakes, potatoes, meat and non-alcoholic beverages (MacLeod et al., 1975).

Magnesium is lost through the gut and in the urine but not, as is the case with potassium, in the sweat. None the less, in severe burns, magnesium is lost in the exudate and severe depletion can occur. Deficiency also results from prolonged gastrointestinal aspiration, severe diarrhoea, gastrointestinal fistulae and in malabsorption, chronic pyelonephritis, hyperaldosteronism and diuretic therapy. Deficiency also follows poor intake in self-neglect, in cirrhosis of the liver (particularly where this is alcoholic in origin) and in malignant disease (Heeley et al., 1974).

The symptoms of magnesium lack are confusion, tremor, ataxia, irritability, weakness and epilepsy. Tetany also occurs if calcium depletion coexists. Diagnosis is certain if the serum magnesium level falls below 0·7 mmol/l, but can exist with normal serum levels, in which case balance studies are required (Whitby et al., 1977).

Treatment of magnesium depletion is by giving magnesium sulphate 1 g of which contains 4 mmol of magnesium. The oral route can be used in non-urgent cases when 1–6 g daily in divided doses is satisfactory. However, purgation frequently results with consequential further loss. The intravenous route is suitable and safe, provided the rate of infusion does not exceed 0·5 mmol/min (Sleisenger, 1963). As much as a litre of 0·5 per cent solution can be given in 24 hours if this rule is observed.

Hypermagnesaemia occurs when the serum level rises about 1 mmol/l in most individuals, but may remain asymptomatic until levels as high as 2·5 mmol/l are reached. Vomiting, weakness, respiratory depression and impairment of consciousness occur. Hypermagnesaemia occurs in chronic renal failure, in the acute stages of renal failure, as a result of giving magnesium salts to patients suffering from subthyroidism or uraemia, and in adrenal failure. Spontaneous recovery results when magnesium intake is stopped when this is the cause, provided renal function is adequate. In an emergency, time may be borrowed by giving intravenously 10–20 ml of 10 per cent calcium gluconate solution over 5–10 minutes, but when as so often is the case, renal function is impaired, dialysis will be required.

REFERENCES
Alberti K. G. M. M., Hockaday T. D. R. and Turner R. C. (1973) *Lancet* **2**, 515.
Allison S. P., Morley C. J. and Burns-Cox C. J. (1972) *Br. Med. J.* **3**, 657.
Burr M. L., St. Leger A. S., Westlake C. A. et al. (1975) *Age Ageing* **4**, 148.
Cowan N. R. and Judge T. G. (1969) *Gerontol. Clin. (Basel)* **13**, 221.
Cox J. R., Horrocks P., Speight C. J. et al. (1971) *Clin. Sci. Mol. Med.* **41**, 55.
Crocket G. S. (1970) *Br. Med. J.* **1**, 171.
Dall J. L. C., Paulose S. and Ferguson J. A. (1971) *Gerontol. Clin. (Basel)* **13**, 114.
Davidson S., Passmore R. and Brock J. F. (1973) *Human Nutrition and Diabetics.* London, Churchill Livingstone.

Davies L. (1973) *Mod. Geriatr.* 3, 482.
Gaddum J. H. (1959) *Pharmacology.* London, Oxford University Press.
Heeley D. M., Warner G. T. and Mayer A. L. R. (1974) *Lancet* 1, 634.
Ibrahim I. K., Ritch A. E. S., MacLennan W. J. (1978) *Age Ageing* 7, 165.
Judge T. G. (1968) *Gerontol. Clin. (Basel)* 10, 102.
Judge T. G. (1969) *Lancet* 2, 221.
Judge T. G. (1973) *Scott. Med. J.* 18, 121.
Judge T. G., Caird F. I., Leask R. G. S. et al. (1974) *Age Ageing* 3, 167.
Judge T. G. and Macleod C. (1968) *5th Europ. Meeting of Clinical Gerontol.* Brussels, p. 295.
Kaul A., Jekat F. and Starlinger H. (1965) *Int. Z. Angew. Physiol.* 21, 62.
Lawson D. H., Murray R. M. and Parker J. L. W. (1972) *Q. J. Med.* 41, 1.
Leask R. G. S., Andrews G. R. and Caird F. I. (1973) *Age Ageing* 2, 14.
MacLennan W. J., Lye M. D. W. and May T. (1977) *Age Ageing* 6, 46.
MacLeod C., Judge T. G. and Caird F. I. (1975) *Age Ageing* 4, 49.
Morgenstern L., Freilich M. and Panish J. F. (1965) *J. Am. Med. Assoc.* 191, 637.
NAS/NRC (1964) (*see* General References).
Pick A. (1966) *Am. Heart J.* 72, 295.
Robson J. S. (1974) In: MacLeod J. (ed.), *Davidson's Principles and Practice of Medicine.* London, Churchill Livingstone.
Sleisenger M. H. (1963) In: Beeson P. B. and MacDermott W. W. B. (ed.) *Cecil-Loeb Textbook of Medicine,* 11th ed. Philadelphia, Saunders.
Whitby L. G., Percy-Robb I. W. and Smith A. F. (1977) *Lecture Notes in Clinical Chemistry.* Oxford, Blackwell Scientific Publications.
Zilva J. and Pannall P. R. (1975) *Clinical Chemistry in Diagnosis and Treatment.* London, Lloyd-Luke.

5. TRACE ELEMENTS
M. H. N. Golden

Of the 95 naturally occurring elements no less than 24 perform essential functions in the body and must be supplied in the diet. Fourteen of these (iron, zinc, manganese, copper, cobalt, molybdenum, chromium, nickel, vanadium, tin, iodine, selenium, fluorine and silicon) are required in very small amounts and are usually referred to as the trace elements.

Unlike the macroelements, whose functions and requirements have received a great deal of attention, the roles that the trace elements play have only been adequately elucidated for iron, iodine and cobalt (in vitamin B_{12}): these are considered in Chapters 10 and 15. The evidence for the importance of the other trace elements is largely drawn from work with experimental animals, and their relevance to the disease of the elderly is circumstantial but tantalizing.

FUNCTIONS OF TRACE ELEMENTS
The trace elements are all highly reactive chemically. Most exist in more than one valency state. They are at the active sites of nearly half the body's enzymes and act both at the catalytic site and to maintain the tertiary structure of proteins (Riordan and Vallee, 1973). It is little wonder that they are nutritionally important. All the trace elements bind strongly to proteins and other ligands, with only minute fractions in the free state. They readily take part in reactions to form organic complexes. The metabolism of these reactive elements is closely controlled within the body, with specific transport and binding proteins. They are strictly compartmentalized both between and within tissues.

ABSORPTION
The metallic elements are homeostatically controlled primarily through their absorption from the intestine (Sahagian et al., 1971) and most undergo an enterohepatic circulation; there is little renal excretion. The actual availability from the diet is dependent upon the particular ligand or complex that happens to bind the element in the diet. For example, the availability of chromium varies from up to 25 per cent from organic complexes (Mertz and Roginski, 1971) to less than 1 per cent for inorganic chromium (Donaldson and Barreras, 1966). If the gross content of a diet is inadequate, deficiency can be predicted. However, if there are chelating

agents in the diet, the metal may be almost totally unavailable, so that a diet with a normal content cannot be presumed to provide adequate trace element nutrition. In fact human zinc deficiency as found in Iran occurs despite gross intakes which are often in excess of those in the West (Reinhold et al., 1973). Plant fibre and phytate are chelating agents which reduce metal availability (Oberleas and Harland, 1977).

The non-metallic trace elements are usually well absorbed and are controlled by renal excretion.

TRACE ELEMENT INTERACTIONS

Apart from chelation, trace element metabolism may be profoundly affected by interaction with other trace elements. They share binding proteins and often fall into similar chemical groups which undergo similar chemical reactions. These interactions potentially involve any pair of elements, essential or non-essential, so that the number of possible interactions is enormous. Only a few have been examined, some of which are show in *Table* 5.1 (Davies, 1974; Suttle, 1975). The magnitude of the effect that these interactions may have is illustrated by a diet of given copper content being either toxic or deficient (for cattle) depending upon the molybdenum and sulphate content (Suttle, 1974). None of the trace elements can be considered in isolation. We have induced copper deficiency with zinc supplementation in children (unpublished) and adults (Porter et al., 1977). The effects of imbalance should be carefully considered in any supplementation programme or treatment.

ASSESSMENT OF TRACE ELEMENT STATUS

If a patient's status of a trace element is to be precisely measured, it is necessary to know the most vulnerable functional site of the element, at that time and in that patient, and to be able to identify the metabolically active fraction of the total pool of the element. Measurement of blood cobalt cannot be used to assess vitamin B_{12} status, though haemoglobin and thyroxine are used to measure iron and iodine status. For these latter elements the functional sites and active fractions are known and measured, not the gross elemental content. With the other elements the functional sites and metabolically active fractions are not known with any certainty. Thus, of necessity, one must rely on direct assay of the gross concentration of the element in an accessible tissue. The results obtained are often cited and acted on as evidence of deficiency. We should be aware of the limitations of these measurements, as will be illustrated with reference to zinc. Plasma contains less than 1 per cent of body zinc. Since zinc like all trace elements is predominantly intracellular, a relatively small shift in body zinc may lead to large plasma concentration changes. Thus a low plasma zinc is found not only in zinc deficiencies but also in infections, trauma, myocardial infarction, neoplasms and even low dose oestrogen therapy (Halsted and Smith, 1970). Obviously a low plasma zinc must be

Table 5.1. Interactions Between Trace Elements

Mechanism	Iron	Iodine	Copper	Zinc	Molybdenum	Selenium	Chromium	Manganese
Unknown	Lead Cobalt	Arsenic Cobalt Manganese	Lead Mercury Nickel	Selenium Iron Nickel	?	Copper Mercury Cadmium Tellurium	Cadmium Vanadium Nickel Zirconium	Calcium Cadmium Nickel
Forms unavailable complexes	Phosphorus Calcium Sulphur	?	Phosphorus Calcium Sulphur Molybdenum	Phosphorus Calcium Sulphur	?	Arsenic		Phosphorus Calcium Sulphur
Competitive inhibition in metabolic pathways	Manganese Cobalt	?	Cadmium Silver Zinc	Cadmium Copper	Sulphur Tungsten	Sulphur	?	Iron
Alteration of metal binding proteins	Zinc Cadmium	?	Cadmium Zinc Molybdenum	Cadmium Mercury	Copper	?	?	?
Changes in enzyme metal complex	?	?	Zinc Molybdenum	Copper	Copper	?	?	?
Alteration in excretion	Copper	?	Molybdenum	?	Sulphur Copper	Arsenic	?	?

interpreted with caution. Total tissue zinc is little better, for an animal can die from experimental zinc deficiency without much change in the gross tissue content (Williams and Mills, 1970). Hair has been extensively used to measure zinc status (Klevay, 1970). However, although the concentration falls with decreasing intake, with further dietary zinc restriction it rises from a nadir because of reduced hair growth (Pallauf and Kirchgessner, 1973) (*Fig.* 5.1). The human counterpart is the low hair zinc, which is

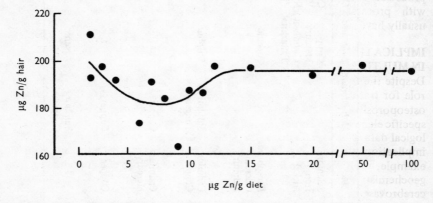

Fig. 5.1. The relationship between the zinc content of the diet and the concentration of zinc in rat hair. $y = 215 - 11x + 1{\cdot}12x^2 - 0{\cdot}031x^3$, $R = 0{\cdot}24$, $P{<}0{\cdot}05$. [Redrawn from data of Pallauf and Kirchgessner (1973).]

found in mild zinc deficiency (Hambidge et al., 1972) but not in severe deficiency (Bradfield et al., 1969). A therapeutic response to supplementation is the only reliable measure of deficiency at present.

There is an extensive literature on tissue levels of trace elements, often showing massive changes and redistribution in disease, particularly degenerative disease. The mechanisms underlying these changes are quite unknown. Although suggestive of deficiency a gross reduction without measurement of the relevant pool or function is difficult to evaluate in clinical terms.

IMPORTANCE OF DEFICIENCIES

Without being able to measure trace metal status or requirements, many authorities thought it unlikely that deficiencies of trace metals would occur in humans, despite the existing well known examples of iron and iodine. Since the profound effects of the biological chelating agents upon availability and elemental interactions on metabolism have been demonstrated, the likelihood of human deficiency has been realized, and patients found who respond to therapeutic trials of zinc, copper and chromium. Subsequently tentative recommended daily allowances of 15 mg zinc and 2 mg copper have been made (NAS/NRC, 1974; Harper, 1977). Unfortunately we do not know the requirements with any precision in normal man, let alone how they are altered by ageing and disease.

The elderly are a vulnerable group in whom all the expected circumstances leading to deficiency exist. They have a restricted diet both in terms of variety and amount of food with a greater use of convenience and processed foods (*see* Chapter 7). Large losses of trace elements occur with processing (Shroeder, 1971), and vegetable protein substitutes usually have significant chelating properties (Oberleas and Harland, 1977).

IMPLICATIONS FOR A ROLE FOR TRACE METAL INVOLVEMENT IN MULTIFACTORIAL DISEASES

Despite the difficulties with trace element assessment there is evidence of a role for trace metal involvement in hypertension, diabetes, atherosclerosis, osteoporosis and rheumatoid arthritis. These will be considered under the specific elements concerned. Beside the specific data must be put epidemiological data which relate diseases to the geochemical environment, with the implication that mineral elements are involved in the aetiology. For example, multiple sclerosis has been related to copper and molybdenum geochemistry (Layton and Sutherland, 1975), and cardiovascular and cerebrovascular deaths to the water supply.

The Water Factor

Over twenty years ago Kobayashi (1957) showed that mortality from stroke was directly related to the acidity of local river water. This observation has led to over thirty studies which attempt to characterize the factors involved. Most of these studies have found factors in reservoir water which correlate with death rates from various vascular diseases. Several studies have failed to find a relationship (Lindeman and Assenzo, 1964; Allwright et al., 1974; Mulcahy, 1964). The most convincing evidence comes from two studies where a change in a local supply led to a change in mortality rate from vascular disease in the British Isles (Crawford et al., 1971), and in the Florida Keys, where there was a drop in cardiac death rate when hard water was introduced from the mainland followed by an increase when the water was artificially softened (Groover et al., 1972).

Hardness of water represents a geochemical mixture of at least 20 elements. In the 30 studies some 36 different variables have been found to correlate with some form of arterial disease. The difficulties with this type of approach are enormous with differences in death certification accuracy and practice as well as those caused by sampling municipal water rather than consumed water. None of the reports implicating individual components is convincing.

It is rarely appreciated that in general less than 10 per cent of one's daily trace element intake is derived from the waterworks. It is unlikely that variation within this 10 per cent will be critical. Perhaps Kobayashi's original paper, where acidity was emphasized, gives the clue. The corrosiveness of water is related inversely to its hardness (Schroeder and Kraemer, 1974). Large amounts of copper, lead, cadmium, zinc and antimony may be picked up from domestic pipes and storage tanks, so that the water actually consumed may give the major body burden of these metals.

It is unlikely that further epidemiological studies of local water supplies will shed light on the problem. We must develop and test mechanistic hypotheses to explain how the elements concerned cause vascular disease.

CHELATING AGENTS

A further area of circumstantial evidence implicating trace elements in degenerative disease is the therapeutic use of chelating agents. Many drugs bind strongly to metals and lead to their elimination. Tetracycline, for example, may lead to the total unavailability of iron and vice versa (Neuvonen et al., 1970). Nearly all the antihypertensive drugs that act by lowering peripheral resistance (e.g. hydralazine) are chelating agents as are many of the psychotropic and anxiolytic agents. This aspect of drug action warrants more thorough investigation.

Of great interest is the circumstantial evidence that in rheumatoid arthritis there is abnormal trace metal metabolism. Gold therapy has long been known to be effective; penicillamine, a strong chelating agent for transition metals, is also effective (Andrews et al., 1973) and zinc sulphate has recently been shown to alleviate symptoms (Simkin, 1976).

ZINC

Unlike iron, where the major body load is in a single protein in a single tissue, zinc occurs in substantial amounts in many tissues of the body. The retina, prostate, Paneth cells and pancreatic islets are exceptionally rich in zinc. Zinc occurs in over 70 enzymes involved in all major metabolic pathways (Riordan and Vallee, 1976). Many of the enzymes involved in protein, RNA and DNA synthesis are zinc metallo-enzymes, as are aldolases, phosphatases and dehydrogenases. Abnormalities of protein synthesis are a constant finding in experimental zinc deficiency.

Apart from its role in enzymes, zinc is important in two other respects. Firstly it modulates the functions of biomembranes, stabilizing lysosomal, mitochondrial, neurotubular and cell membranes (Chvapil, 1973) and altering the activity of the sodium pump (Patrick et al., 1978b). Secondly zinc protects against both lipid peroxidation (Chvapil et al., 1972) and free radical formation (Willson, 1977). These toxic products are formed in tissue from oxygen catalysed by iron or copper. Vitamin E and selenium (glutathione peroxidase) act by reducing the peroxides formed, and zinc is thought to act by itself combining with the organic precursors of peroxides and free radicals and displacing iron or copper. This is potentially the most important function of bound zinc, as free radicals and lipid peroxides have been implicated in the aetiology of ageing (Witting, 1977) and carcinoma (Wattenberg et al., 1976).

Zinc is unique amongst the trace metals in that there is no functional body store of zinc. Rats on a zinc-deficient diet for several days begin to show signs of deficiency (Williams and Mills, 1970) and a zinc-deficient diet for three days is a potent teratogen (Hurley and Swenerton, 1971) even preimplantation embryos are susceptible to acute deficiency (Hurley and Shrader, 1975). We do not yet know the critical pools of zinc in determining the hierarchy and rapidity of onset of symptoms. Nevertheless, it is clear that zinc deficiency may supervene very rapidly in humans. Zinc, by virtue of its key role in protein and nucleic acid synthesis, is needed to replace lost tissue. Pories et al. (1967a, b) studied fit healthy patients undergoing surgery for pilonidal sinus operations: zinc supplementation led to healing of the wound at more than twice the rate of the unsupplemented group. This is the counterpart of the animal studies which showed no body store of zinc. In the face of an increased demand for zinc to synthesize new tissue, these previously healthy servicemen did not have sufficient zinc in their diets. Zinc-rich diets must be given when healing is required. These results have been confirmed in healing of burned skin (Larsen et al., 1970), arterial ischaemic ulceration (Haeger and Lanner, 1974), and chronic venous ulceration (Husaine, 1969; Greaves and Skillen, 1970; Serjeant et al., 1970, Hallböök and Lanner, 1972). That this is not a pharmacological effect of zinc is shown by the failure to show improvement in healing when the diet is sufficient in zinc (Pories and Strain, 1974). Poor healing is common in the elderly. Where ununited fractures, ulcers and bed sores are found a trial of zinc should be considered.

The diets of the elderly are frequently deficient in total zinc content both in institutions (Greger, 1977) and at home (Greger and Sciscoe, 1977; Abdulla et al., 1977). This inadequate intake is reflected in the decreasing plasma zinc with age in some populations (Lindeman et al., 1971; Chooi et al., 1976) and also in decreasing bone zinc with age (Alhava et al., 1977). Bone zinc is thought to be a reasonable measure of zinc nutrition (Momčilović et al., 1975). The elderly as a group are found to have a high proportion of low plasma zincs (Hallböök and Hedelin, 1977; Tengrup and Samuelsson, 1977; Vir and Love, 1979). These studies taken in conjunction indicate that zinc deficiency is a frequent finding in the elderly population.

The classic signs and symptoms of zinc deficiency are dwarfism and hypogonadism (Halsted et al., 1974), and are thus of course not found in the elderly, in whom the signs and symptoms of zinc deficiency are delayed wound healing and skin ulceration. Anorexia is a constant feature of nearly all patients with zinc deficiency (Halsted et al., 1974). Abnormalities and perversions of the sense of smell and taste are frequent (Henkin et al., 1974, 1976) and may respond to zinc in the elderly (Greger and Geissler, 1978). Zinc-deficient patients have thin atrophic skin, poor hair and nail growth and abnormalities of vitamin A metabolism leading to night blindness (Morrison et al., 1978). Zinc deficiency also leads to a defective cell-mediated immune response (Golden et al., 1978a), so that infections with organisms normally considered as commensals are common in zinc deficiency. We have recently skin tested 5 elderly patients with chronic mucocutaneous candidiasis, only temporarily suppressed by nystatin therapy, using Candida antigen, with and without zinc supplementation. In each case zinc enhanced the reaction to the antigen, and systemic treatment with zinc led to a clearance of the candidiasis (Golden et al., 1978b). The occurrence of Candida infections and intertrigo should lead to an investigation of zinc status.

A syndrome of acute zinc deficiency in adults treated with the chelating agent histidine (Henkin et al., 1975) was associated with bizarre psychiatric disturbances, responsive to zinc therapy.

Zinc deficiency occurs secondarily to numerous diseases (Sandstead et al., 1977). The signs of zinc deficiency, although far from unique to zinc deficiency, are common in the elderly. Zinc deficiency is probably far more common than is generally realized.

COPPER

Unlike zinc, copper has not yet been shown to be deficient in any substantial population. Nevertheless evidence is accumulating to show that copper deficiency may be more prevalent than is currently thought. The diets of two decades ago had adequate copper in them, but with the replacement of copper pipes, tanks and cooking vessels with plastic and aluminium, together with the increasing use of refined foods, many modern diets do not meet the recommended dietary intake of 2 mg per day (Klevay, 1977).

Anaemia is the classic feature of copper deficiency. It is caused by an inability to transport iron to the bone marrow. Iron can only be transported on transferrin in the ferric state, yet it is absorbed and stored in the ferrous state. The enzyme responsible for oxidizing the iron prior to transport is the copper-containing circulating protein caeruloplasmin. A deficiency of copper thus leads to loss of ferroxidase activity and anaemia (Osaki et al., 1971; Frieden and Hsieh, 1976).

Animals on a copper-deficient diet may die from arterial aneurysms (Coulson and Carnes, 1963). This is due to defective cross-linking of the proelastin and procollagen molecules. These cross-links are formed from adjacent lysine residues condensing to form desmosine. The lysyl oxidase that catalyses this reaction is a copper metallo-enzyme (Chou et al., 1970). To my knowledge this enzyme and copper nutrition have not been assessed in patients with aneurysmal disease, or defects in collagen formation. Copper-deficient children have osteoporosis probably due to defective collagen biosynthesis (Ashkenazi et al., 1973). Copper nutrition and interaction should be examined in the elderly from this viewpoint.

Copper deficiency in animals may lead to ataxia and paralysis. The brains of these animals have a deficiency of three copper metallo-enzymes, cytochrome C-oxidase, superoxide dismutase, and dopamine-hydroxylase (Prohaska and Wells, 1974) involved in energy supply, superoxide protection and neurotransmitter synthesis. There are many similarities between copper deficiency and both manganese toxicity and Parkinson's disease (O'Dell et al., 1976). Copper deficiency has been implicated in both atherogenesis (Klevay, 1977) and protection from atheroma (Harman, 1968); the position is unclear.

CHROMIUM

Animals fed a diet deficient in chromium develop glycosuria, fasting hyperglycaemia, hypercholesterolaemia, corneal opacities and aortic plaques (Davidson and Blackwell, 1968; Schroeder, 1968). The similarity of these consistent and reproducible effects to human diabetes is remarkable.

For activity chromium has to be incorporated into an organic complex. This complex is a tetra-aqua-dinicotinate with glycine, glutamic acid and cysteine bound at the coordination sites (Mertz et al., 1974). It has been designated glucose tolerance factor (GTF) and *in vitro* it potentiates every action of insulin (Mertz, 1969). *In vivo* it is metabolized entirely differently from inorganic chromium, being concentrated in the liver, and crossing the placenta actively (Gürson, 1977).

Unfortunately there is neither a precise assay for GTF nor a supply of pure GTF for clinical evaluation (Mertz). Even the assay of chromium itself is extremely difficult. Preparation can lead to losses of volatile chromium (Maxia et al., 1972) and contamination is surprisingly easy, so much so that values for plasma chromium in the literature differ by up to an order of magnitude (Hambidge, 1974).

Despite these difficulties the chromium content of tissues has been shown to decrease steadily with advancing age (Schroeder et al., 1962) and with successive pregnancies (Hambidge, 1971). Furthermore, hair chromium is much lower in patients with diabetes mellitus (Hambidge et al., 1968; Benjanuvatra and Bennion, 1975). Normal subjects have an increase in blood chromium with a glucose load (Mertz et al., 1974) followed by an increase in urinary chromium excretion. Diabetic subjects fail to show this increase in blood or urinary chromium after a glucose load (Gürson, 1977). In this context it is of interest that Cranfield and Doisy (1976) demonstrated a correlation between increasing age and decreased urinary chromium excretion.

There have been a number of therapeutic trials of inorganic chromium salts in patients with impaired glucose tolerance. Despite the fact that unphysiological forms of chromium have been used there has been, in general, an improvement in glucose tolerance with long term treatment (Glinsman and Mertz, 1966; Levine et al., 1968; Schroeder, 1968). The studies were not blind and involved small numbers of patients. One study used brewer's yeast supplements which had a high content of GTF and a marked improvement was found (Doisy et al., 1977).

The evidence that chromium deficiency is a factor in atherosclerosis is even more tenuous at the moment. It consists of low levels of chromium in the aorta of patients with cardiovascular disease (Schroeder et al., 1970) and elevated cholesterol and plaques in animals on a chromium-deficient diet (Schroeder and Balassa, 1965). One study has shown no difference between the urinary chromium excretion of atherosclerotic patients and normal patients (Punsar et al., 1977).

Until the biologically active forms of chromium can be readily and precisely assayed, and are available for large scale, blind, therapeutic trial, it will not be possible to fully evaluate the role of chromium in these diseases, that are so common in the elderly.

CADMIUM

Administering cadmium in low doses (but not high doses) to rats induces hypertension (Perry et al., 1977a, b). The histological changes in the hypertensive animals are similar to those in hypertensive humans (Kanisawa and Schroeder, 1969) and can be treated by administering zinc, the biological antagonist of cadmium (Schroeder et al., 1968). These animal studies have led to a number of investigations in man, with conflicting results. Cadmium concentrations have been found to be elevated in human hypertensive kidneys (Schroeder and Vinton, 1962; Lener and Bibr, 1971) and blood (Glauser et al., 1976; Thind and Fisher, 1976). Other studies have failed to confirm these findings in kidneys (Syversen et al., 1976; Østergaard, 1977) and blood (Wester, 1973; Beevers et al., 1976). There are a number of explanations for these discrepancies. Some authors failed to take smoking into account, a factor which increases tissue cadmium levels. The narrow dose-response curve reported by Perry et al. (1977b) may be important. The interaction of trace metals has not been considered. Adequate zinc intake protects against cadmium toxicity (Vigliani, 1969; Fox, 1974). It is noteworthy that the studies with positive responses originated in the USA, where zinc intake is particularly suspect. Indeed Thind and Fisher (1974) showed that a low plasma zinc was associated with hypertension. A further interaction of importance seems to be that with selenium. Hypertension does not occur if the cadmium is dissolved in hard water or in water with a high selenium content (Perry et al., 1974). The role of cadmium would be easier to assess if the mechanisms by which cadmium raised the blood pressure were known. In this regard cadmium increases plasma renin levels (Perry and Erlanger, 1973), augments the pressor activity of kidney homogenates (Maier et al., 1974) and causes sodium retention (Doyle et al., 1975). Hypertensive patients have an impairment of the sodium pump in their white cells which reverts to normal with treatment (Edmondson et al., 1975). In arterioles from animals with experimental hypertension there is also impairment of the sodium pump (Overbeck et al., 1976). The white cell sodium pump is stimulated by zinc (Patrick et al., 1978a) and probably the red cell pump also (Swaminathan et al., 1976). The sodium pump is inhibited by cadmium (Patrick et al., 1978a). It is possible that cadmium may cause hypertension by inhibiting the arteriolar sodium pump leading to partial depolarization and increased vascular resistance. The precise role that cadmium plays in human essential hypertension must await further studies.

OTHER TRACE ELEMENTS

We are even more ignorant about the metabolic functions and relationship to disease of the other trace elements. Experimental depletion or toxicity in animals has shown many interesting relationships. Selenium deficiency predisposes to superoxide liver damage, cataracts, hair loss and pancreatic degeneration (Burk, 1977). Manganese is essential for mucopolysaccharide synthesis and deficiency produces chondrodystrophy (Leach, 1971); manganese salts can reverse hydralazine-induced disseminated lupus erythematosus (Comens, 1956). Silicon seems to have a role in cross-linkage within connective tissue (Nielsen and Sandstead, 1974). Almost all the trace elements affect cholesterol metabolism. With none of these is there direct evidence for involvement in the diseases of the elderly.

SUMMARY

Circumstantial evidence is accumulating to suggest that deficiencies of zinc, copper and chromium and an excess of cadmium may be particularly prevalent in our geriatric population. These trace metals are implicated in most of the major degenerative diseases; however the precise role of these elements is uncertain. The therapeutic alteration of the dietary intake of trace elements or manipulation of their metabolism is likely to be of great importance in the future.

ACKNOWLEDGEMENTS
I thank Drs Barbara Golden and Alan Jackson for many stimulating conversations, the Wellcome Trust for support, and my patients for showing me the power of these micronutrients.

REFERENCES
Abdulla M., Jägerstad M., Nordén A. et al. (1977) *Nutr. Metab.* **21**, Suppl. 1, 41.
Alhava E. M., Olkkonen H., Puittinen J. et al. (1977) *Acta Orthop. Scand.* **48**, 1.
Allwright S. P., Coulson A., Detels R. et al. (1974) *Lancet* **1**, 860.
Andrews F. M., Golding D. N., Freeman A. M. et al. (1973) *Lancet* **1**, 275.
Ashkenazi A., Levin S., Djaldetti M. et al. (1973) *Paediatrics* **52**, 525.
Beevers D. G., Campbell B. C., Goldberg A. et al. (1976) *Lancet* **2**, 1222.
Benjanuvatra N. K. and Bennion M. (1975) *Nutr. Rep. Int.* **12**, 325.
Bradfield R. B., Yee T. and Baertl J. M. (1969) *Am. J. Clin. Nutr.* **22**, 1349.
Burk R. F. (1977) In: Prasad A. S. (ed.), (*see* General References) p. 105.
Chooi M. K., Todd J. K. and Boyd N. D. (1976) *Nutr. Metabol.* **20**, 135.

Chou W. S., Rucker R. B., Savage J. E. et al. (1970) *Proc. Soc. Exp. Biol. Med.* **134**, 1078.

Chvapil M. (1973) *Life Sci.* **13**, 1041.

Chvapil M., Peng V. M., Aronson A. L. et al. (1972) *J. Nutr.* **104**, 434.

Comens P. (1956) *Am. J. Med.* **20**, 944.

Coulson W. F. and Carnes W. H. (1963) *Am. J. Pathol.* **43**, 945.

Cranfield W. K. and Doisy R. J. (1976) In: Hsu J. M., Davis R. L. and Nerthamer R. W. (ed.), *Biomedical Role of Trace Elements in Aging*. St. Petersburg, Florida, Eckerd College Gerontology Center, p. 117.

Crawford M. D., Gardner M. J. and Morris J. N. (1971) *Lancet* **2**, 327.

Davidson I. W. F. and Blackwell W. L. (1968) *Proc. Soc. Exp. Biol. Med.* **127**, 66.

Davies N. T. (1974) *Proc. Nutr. Soc.* **33**, 293.

Doisy R. J., Streeten D. H. P., Freiberg J. M. et al. (1977) In: Prasad A. S. (ed.), (*see* General References) p. 79.

Donaldson R. M. and Barreras R. F. (1966) *J. Lab. Clin. Med.* **68**, 484.

Doyle J. J., Bernhoft R. A. and Sandstead H. H. (1975) *J. Lab. Clin. Med.* **86**, 57.

Edmondson R. P. S., Thomas R. D., Hilton P. J. et al. (1975) *Lancet* **1**, 103.

Food and Nutrition Board (1974) *Recommended Dietary Allowances* 8th ed. Washington, Natural History of Sciences.

Fox M. R. S. (1974) *J. Food Sci.* **39**, 321.

Frieden E. and Hsieh H. S. (1976) In: Meister A. (ed.), *Advances in Enzymology and Related Areas of Molecular Biology*, Vol. 44. New York, Wiley, p. 187.

Glauser S. C., Bello C. T. and Glauser E. M. (1976) *Lancet* **1**, 717.

Glinsman W. H. and Mertz W. (1966) *Metabolism* **15**, 510.

Golden M. H. N., Golden B. E., Harland P. S. E. G. et al. (1978a) *Lancet* **1**, 1226.

Golden M. H. N., Golden B. E. and Terry S. (1978b) (Unpublished observation).

Greaves M. W. and Skillen A. W. (1970) *Lancet* **2**, 879.

Greger J. L. (1977) *J. Gerontol.* **32**, 549.

Greger J. L. and Geissler A. H. (1978) *Am. J. Clin. Nutr.* **31**, 633.

Greger J. L. and Sciscoe B. S. (1977) *J. Am. Diet. Assoc.* **70**, 37.

Groover M. E., Antell G. E., Fulghum J. E. et al. (1972) *Death Rates following a Sudden Change in Hardness of Drinking Water*. Presented at SER meeting Feb. 28, Tampa, Florida.

Gürson C. T. (1977) In: Draper H. M. (ed.), *Advances in Nutritional Research*, Vol. 1. New York, Plenum, p. 23.

Haeger K. and Lanner E. (1974) *J. Vasc. Dis.* **3**, 77.

Hallböök T. and Hedelin H. (1977) *Br. J. Surg.* **64**, 271.

Hallböök L. T. and Lanner E. (1972) *Lancet* **2**, 780.

Halsted J. A. and Smith J. C. (1970) *Lancet* **1**, 322.

Halsted J. A., Smith J. C. and Irwin M. I. (1974) *J. Nutr.* **104**, 345.

Hambidge K. M. (1971) In: Mertz W. and Cornatzer W. E. (ed.), *Newer Trace Elements in Nutrition*. New York, Dekker, p. 169.

Hambidge K. M. (1974) *Am. J. Clin. Nutr.* **27**, 505.

Hambidge K. M., Hambidge C., Jacobs M. et al. (1972) *Pediatr. Res.* **6**, 868.

Hambidge K. M., Rogerson D. O. and O'Brien D. (1968) *Diabetes* **17**, 517.

Harman D. (1968) *Circulation* **38**, Suppl. 4. 8 (*abstract*).

Harper A. E. (1977) In: Prasad A. S. (ed.), (*see* General References) p. 371.

Henkin R. I., Patten B. M., Re P. K. et al. (1975) *Arch. Neurol.* **32**, 745.

Henkin R. I., Schecter P. J., Friedewald W. T. et al. (1976) *Am. J. Med. Sci.* **272**, 286.

Henkin R. I., Schecter P. J., Raff M. S. et al. (1974) In: Pories et al. (*see* General References) p. 243.

Hurley L. S. and Shrader R. E. (1975) *Nature* **254**, 427.

Hurley L. S. and Swenerton H. (1971) *J. Nutr.* **101**, 597.

Husaine S. L. (1969) *Lancet* **1**, 1069.
Kanisawa M. and Schroeder H. A. (1969) *Exp. Mol. Pathol.* **10**, 81.
Klevay L. M. (1970) *Am. J. Clin. Nutr.* **23**, 284.
Klevay L. M. (1977) In: Draper H. H. (ed.), *Advances in Nutritional Research* Vol. 1. New York, Plenum, p. 227.
Kobayashi K. (1957) *Ber. Ohara Inst. Landw. Biol.* **11**, 12.
Larsen D. L., Maxwell R., Abston S. et al. (1970) *Plast. Reconstr. Surg.* **46**, 13.
Layton W. and Sutherland J. M. (1975) *Med. J. Aust.* **1**, 73.
Leach R. M. (1971) *Fed. Proc.* **30**, 991.
Lener J. and Bibr B. (1971) *Lancet* **1**, 970.
Levine R. A., Streeten D. H. P. and Doisy R. J. (1968) *Metabolism* **17**, 114.
Lindeman R. D. and Assenzo J. R. (1964) *Am. J. Public Health* **54**, 1071.
Lindeman R. D., Clarke M. L. and Colmore J. P. (1971) *J. Gerontol.* **26**, 358.
Maier G. D., Kusiak J. W., Higgins G. L. et al. (1974) *Arch. Environ. Health* **29**, 110.
Maxia V., Meloni S., Rollier M. A. et al. (1972) In: *Nuclear Activation Techniques in the Life Sciences.* Vienna, IAEA, p. 527.
Mertz W. Personal communication.
Mertz W. (1969) *Physiol. Rev.* **49**, 163.
Mertz W. and Roginski E. E. (1971) In: Mertz W. and Cornatzer W. E. (ed.), *Newer Trace Elements in Nutrition.* New York, Dekker, p. 125.
Mertz W., Toepfer E. W., Roginski E. E. et al. (1974) *Fed. Proc.* **33**, 2275.
Momčilović B., Belonje B. and Shah B. G. (1975) *Nutr. Rep. Int.* **11**, 445.
Morrison S. A., Russell R. M., Carney E. A. et al. (1978) *Am. J. Clin. Nutr.* **31**, 276.
Mulcahy R. (1964) *J. Irish Med. Assoc.* **55**, 17.
NAS/NRC (1974) (*see* General References).
Neuvonen P. J., Gothoni G., Hackman R. et al. (1970) *Br. Med. J.* **4**, 532.
Nielsen F. H. and Sandstead H. H. (1974) *Am. J. Clin. Nutr.* **27**, 515.
Oberleas D. and Harland B. F. (1977) In: Brewer G. J. and Prasad A. S. (ed.), *Zinc Metabolism: Current Aspects in Health and Disease.* New York, Liss, p. 11.
O'Dell B. L., Smith R. M. and King R. A. (1976) *J. Neurochem.* **26**, 451.
Osaki S., Johnson D. A. and Frieden E. (1971) *J. Biol. Chem.* **246**, 3018.
Østergaard K. (1977) *Lancet* **1**, 677.
Overbeck H. W., Pamnani M. B., Akera T. et al. (1976) *Circulation Res.* **38**, Suppl. 11, 48.
Pallauf J. and Kirchgessner M. (1973) *Zentralbl. Veterinaermed.* [A] **20**, 100.
Patrick J., Golden M. H. N. and Golden B. E. (1978a) Unpublished observations.
Patrick J., Michael J., Golden M. H N. et al. (1978b) *Clin. Sci. Mol. Med.* **54**, 585.
Perry H. and Erlanger M. (1973) *J. Lab. Clin. Med.* **82**, 399.
Perry H. M. and Perry E. F. (1977d) *Proc. Soc. Exp. Biol. Med.* **156**, 173.
Perry H. M., Erlanger M. and Perry E. F. (1977) *Am. J. Physiol.* **232**, H114.
Perry H. M., Perry E. F., Erlanger M. (1974) In: Hemphill D. D. (ed.), *Trace Substances in Environmental Health.* Columbia, University of Missouri, p. 51.
Pories W. J., Henzel J. H., Rob C. G. et al. (1967a) *Lancet* **1**, 121.
Pories W. J., Henzel J. H., Rob C. G. et al. (1967b) *Ann. Surg.* **165**, 432.
Pories W. J. and Strain W. H. (1974) (*see* General References).
Porter K. G., McMaster D., Elmes M. E. et al. (1977) *Lancet* **2**, 774.
Prohaska J. R. and Wells W. W. (1974) *J. Neurochem.* **23**, 91.
Punsar S., Wolf W., Mertz W. et al. (1977) *Ann. Clin. Res.* **9**, 79.
Reinhold J. G., Nasr K., Lahimgarzadeh A. et al. (1973) *Lancet* **1**, 283.
Riordan J. F. and Vallee B. L. (1973) In: Friedman M. (ed.), *Protein-Metal Interactions.* New York, Plenum, p. 33.
Riordan J. F. and Vallee B. L. (1976) In: Prasad A. S. (ed.), (*see* General References), p. 227.
Sahagian B. M., Barlow I. H. and Perry H. M. (1971) In: Skoryna S. C. and Wandron-Edwards D. (ed.), *Intestinal Absorption of Metal Irons, Trace Elements and Radionuclides.* Oxford, Pergamon, p. 321.

Sandstead H. H., Vo-Khactu K. P. and Solomons N. (1977) In: Prasad A. S. (ed.), (*see* General References).

Schroeder H. A. (1968) *Am. J. Clin. Nutr.* **21**, 230.

Schroeder H. A. (1971) *Am. J. Clin. Nutr.* **24**, 562.

Schroeder H. A. and Balassa J. J. (1965) *Am. J. Physiol.* **209**, 433.

Schroeder H. A., Balassa J. J. and Tipton I. H. (1962) *J. Chronic Dis.* **15**, 941.

Schroeder H. A. and Kraemer L. K. (1974) *Arch. Environ. Health* **28**, 303.

Schroeder H. A., Nason A. P. and Tipton I. H. (1970) *J. Chronic Dis.* **23**, 123.

Schroeder H. A. and Vinton (1962) *Am. J. Physiol.* **202**, 515.

Serjeant G. R., Galloway R. E. and Gueri M. C. (1970) *Lancet* **2**, 891.

Simkin P. A. (1976) *Lancet* **2**, 538.

Suttle N. F. (1974) *Proc. Nutr. Soc.* **33**, 299.

Suttle N. F. (1975) In: Nicholas D. J. D. and Egan A. R. (ed.), *Trace Elements in Soil−Plant−Animal Systems.* New York, Academic, p. 271.

Swaminathan R., Segall N. H., Chapman C. et al. (1976) *Lancet* **2**, 1382.

Syversen T. L. M., Stray T. K., Syversen G. B. et al. (1976) *Scand. J. Clin. Lab. Invest.* **36**, 251.

Tengrup I. and Samuelsson H. (1977) *Acta Chir. Scand.* **143**, 195.

Thind G. S. and Fisher G. M. (1974) *Clin. Sci. Mol. Med.* **46**, 137.

Thind G. S. and Fisher G. M. (1976) *Clin. Sci. Mol. Med.* **51**, 483.

Vigliani E. C. (1969) *Am. Ind. Hyg. Assoc. J.* **30**, 329.

Vir S. C. and Love A. H. G. (1979) *Am. J. Clin. Nutr.* **32**, 1472.

Wattenberg L. W., Loub W. O., Lam L. K. et al. (1976) *Fed. Proc.* **35**, 1327.

Wester P. O. (1973) *Acta Med. Scand.* **194**, 505.

Williams R. B. and Mills C. F. (1970) *Br. J. Nutr.* **24**, 989.

Willson R. L. (1977) In: *Iron Metabolism. Ciba Foundation Symposium 51,* Amsterdam, North-Holland, p. 331.

Witting L. A. (1977) In: Draper H. H. (ed.), *Advances in Nutritional Research,* Vol. 1. New York, Plenum, p. 189.

6. THE METHODOLOGY OF NUTRITION SURVEYS, WITH EMPHASIS ON DIETARY ASPECTS*
M. M. Disselduff

Nutrition is defined in the Oxford English Dictionary as 'The action or process of supplying, or of receiving nourishment'. This chapter will be devoted to a discussion of the problems, specific to the elderly, of collecting, expressing and interpreting nutritional data — that is, data relating to nourishment.

COLLECTION OF DIETARY DATA
For many years dietary surveys have been carried out in order to estimate the energy and nutrient content of the diets of individuals or groups of individuals. Findings from these surveys have been used together with social, economic and environmental information to confirm, or in part to explain, clinical and laboratory findings. They have also been used as a basis for educational advice. It should be emphasized that dietary surveys alone cannot be used to assess nutritional status. In the final analysis diagnosis of nutritional status is a clinical judgement, although made with the help of laboratory findings and a knowledge of energy and nutrient intakes.

METHODS OF DIETARY ASSESSMENT
All dietary surveys have a common objective — to discover the food intakes of individuals or groups of individuals and to translate these food intakes into energy and nutrients which, in turn, are related to state of health. The degree of precision of the data will depend on the purpose of the survey and the choice of method is therefore determined by the objective.

Four main types of dietary survey are in common use:

1. Dietary histories obtained by interview (Burke, 1947).

2. Recall interviews, usually relating to the previous 24 hours and carried out on one or more occasions (Wiehl, 1942).

3. Weighed dietary records kept over varying periods of time (DHSS, 1972; Lonergan et al., 1975).

4. Chemical analysis of identical samples of food consumed.

*The contents of this chapter represent the author's views alone and in no way commit the Department of Health and Social Security.

Marr (1971) and Young and Trulson (1960) have discussed the strengths and weaknesses of these methods and emphasized the importance of choosing a method appropriate to the objective of the study. It is generally agreed that chemical analysis give the most accurate result but is time-consuming, expensive and difficult; and probably (although this cannot be quantified) introduces an unacceptable degree of bias when used in the community. For practical purposes this method is usually appropriate only in an institutional environment or where very small numbers are involved, and it will not be considered here. Discussion here will be limited to methods used in dietary studies of the elderly living in the community in developed countries.

If dietary intakes are to be related to clinical findings the practical method giving most precision (i.e. method 3, the weighed dietary record) is indicated. If crude information, in qualitative terms, is sufficient a cruder survey method (either method 1, dietary history, or method 2, recall) may suffice. In practice many workers (Exton-Smith and Stanton, 1965; DHSS, 1972; Caird et al., 1975) use modifications of the three basic methods which are, in effect, combinations of two or more of these methods, developed as a result of extensive pilot studies and shown to be workable when the surveyed population is elderly. Attempts are made constantly to refine and simplify methods. MacLeod (1972) and Disselduff (1973) have compared methods using the same subjects. The former concluded that for individuals the 24-hour recall method alone was unlikely to give reliable information; and the latter found no constant relationship between results obtained by the three different methods. However, interpretation of such studies is difficult because of the unknown effect of one method upon others if information is collected simultaneously; and because of the possibility that, if the time lapse between the three studies is of substantial length, differences obtained may in fact be true differences over the period rather than apparent differences due to differences in method. Durnin and Blake (1962) reported the reassuring finding that energy intakes, calculated from weighed dietary records, corresponded within 5 per cent to energy expenditure. It is generally agreed that the quantitative record (however achieved) reinforced by a dietary history is the method of choice when dealing with an elderly population.

FOOD COMPOSITION TABLES

An appropriate food composition table from which to calculate the energy and nutrient content of the diet is a fundamental requirement. No food composition table can do more than offer representative values for different foods – a limitation which is not always appreciated. Widdowson and McCance (1943) made this point when they said: 'There are two schools of thought about food tables. One tends to regard the figures in them as having the accuracy of atomic weight determinations; the other dismisses them as valueless on the ground that a foodstuff may be so modified by the soil, the season or its rate of growth that no figure can be a reliable guide to its composition. The truth of course lies somewhere between these points of view.' The accuracy of the food composition table should be matched by the accuracy of food description, of measurements of foods consumed and of methods of analysis of the data. To combine crude and precise measurements within the one study makes nonsense of results.

If the food composition table is constructed in such a way that foods of similar nutrient content are grouped together it is easier to identify food sources of nutrients, as well as total intakes of foods and nutrients.

DURATION OF DIETARY SURVEYS

If dietary assessment is to be related to clinical findings it is important that the period of the survey should be representative. It is sometimes suggested that the problem of ensuring that dietary information is typical of the normal pattern is less when dealing with the aged. There may be some truth in this but it is a dangerous generalization. Old people are not a homogeneous group. They share one common characteristic – that all have survived beyond the arbitrary age of retirement. In other respects there is as much variation in life style (including eating habits) as can be found in any other age group. Consequently, there is always some doubt as to whether dietary intakes on any single occasion are representative of usual eating patterns.

It is reasonable to assume that the longer the period of the survey the more likely is the record to be representative. However the optimum duration is not known. Neither is it known whether familiarity with the method improves accuracy of recording or whether, after a certain period, it results in carelessness. A seven-day weighed survey is commonly used (Judge et al., 1974 and DHSS, 1972). Repeat studies, conducted at intervals (DHSS, 1972; Disselduff, 1973), while not proving that 7 days are long enough to show normal eating patterns, give some reassurance in that subjects largely fall into the same dietary ranking order on each occasion. Seasonal variations can be detected by making repeat studies at intervals. Such tests of reproducibility are never conclusive since the many variables affecting food consumption cannot be eliminated. Two further checks can be employed: a diet history in conjunction with the weighed record will draw attention to discrepancies between 'usual' meal patterns and the actual record; a 'case history' as used by DHSS (1972) describing the social and physical environment of the respondent at the time of the survey may make it clear whether the week of the study is or is not typical.

COMPARATIVE STUDIES

Comparisons between surveys carried out by the same method and using the same food composition table (DHSS, unpublished) have shown good agreement (MacLeod, 1972; DHSS, 1972). Similarly good agreement has been claimed (Debry et al., 1977) when comparing results from surveys where neither the method nor the food composition table was common to all. A certain amount of caution should be expressed about the latter claim since it is possible that compensating errors are responsible for the apparent agreement.

LONGITUDINAL STUDIES

Nutritional status in old age may be determined partly by the quality of the diet eaten in youth. Reliable quantitative information about food habits cannot be obtained retrospectively. Because of the time interval between under- or over-consumption of energy or nutrients and clinical evidence of deficiency or imbalance, longitudinal studies are much more likely to reveal cause and effect than are cross-sectional studies, although the latter are useful to show present consumption and to indicate individuals or groups of individuals who may be at future risk.

THE HUMAN ELEMENT

Because so many old people suffer from poor eyesight, defective hearing and arthritic hands they may require a great deal of help to keep diet records. MacLeod (1972) and DHSS (1972) report the need for frequent visiting and careful supervision of an appreciable number of the subjects they have surveyed. Essential socio-economic data are collected during the course of the study so even in the absence of mental or physical handicap several visits are necessary. There is always the chance that such intrusion may have an effect on eating habits. This cannot be quantified, but after close association over a period of time the experienced fieldworker should be able to judge whether his presence has interfered with normal meal patterns.

The question of bias is one which worries most workers. It is reasonable to assume that respondents will react in some way to the unfamiliar emphasis placed on food when it is weighed or recorded at the time of consumption. Some may be objective about this, others may be surprised to discover how much (or how little) of a specific food they are eating and may, deliberately, restrict (or increase) amounts. Such changes are unquantifiable. Histories and repeat studies may go some way towards clarifying the situation but the problems of interpretation (as discussed above) remain.

Another form of bias is introduced by the observer. Large scale dietary surveys involve a number of interviewers and therefore there is a possibility of inter-observer variation. Steen (1977) has shown that it is possible to detect some differences between observers and most workers would agree with his conclusion that, where subjective interpretation is required, it is inevitable that there will be differences, however thorough the training. The risk of undetected bias may be greater when only one observer is used.

Because of the inevitably close association between the interviewer and the elderly respondent, the personality as well as the professional competence of the fieldworker is very important. Reference is often made in the literature to 'experienced' or 'competent' interviewers (Davidson et al., 1962) but nowhere are the personal and professional qualifications listed. When the interviewer is responsible, or partly responsible, for planning and interpreting studies in addition to carrying out the fieldwork, professional qualifications in food and nutrition and in research techniques are important; but without the necessary personal qualities these qualifications are of little use. When the interviewer is responsible only for contacting respondents, instructing in the method, supervising and helping in the recording of data and for coding records, professional training is of secondary importance. A housewife's knowledge of foods and weights of foods, together with normal intelligence and an interest in the subject, are the basic requirements. For both types of fieldworker personal characteristics are of paramount importance. The most erudite nutritionist will fail in the field if he is not acceptable to the subject. Tolerance, patience, sensitivity, a sense of humour, understanding and compassion, combined with an objective attitude, are all essential. A patronizing or didactic attitude guarantees rejection. Social conventions can be less important in old age and many old people will express (sometimes quite explicitly) resentment at what they regard as impudent interference. The degree of cooperation and the final response rate depends on the front-line worker.

PRESENTATION OF FINDINGS

The collection of dietary data is not a justifiable end in itself. In isolation it can only mean that a given person or group of persons, at a given time, ate certain foods which contained certain nutrients. It is not possible to state that the consumers gained the benefit of these nutrients – merely that they may have done so. This is particularly true in the case of old people. Disease may inhibit digestion or absorption. Calculated dietary intakes are indicators of the quality of the diet but do not guarantee adequacy or otherwise. Why, then, collect this information? Because, in conjunction with other data, it can contribute to the understanding of clinical and laboratory findings and suggest ways of preventing or curing conditions of nutritional deficiency or excess.

Basic presentation of dietary findings is usually in two forms:

1. As energy and nutrient intakes.

2. As a percentage of total energy and total nutrients contributed by individual foods or groups of foods.

Frequency distributions of these findings reveal much more than mean intakes for groups. Average individual intakes of energy and nutrients, providing they are representative of usual eating patterns, can be related to social, economic, medical and laboratory findings. Average intakes for groups of individuals must be treated more cautiously, because of the probable variation in requirements. Some workers relate mean intakes to figures of recommended intakes of nutrients. This is not a meaningful way to express results. Recommended intakes, to have any meaning, should be based on a knowledge of the range of requirements of a given group of people. Requirements of the elderly are not known with any certainty.

The human body requires energy and nutrients, but the human being eats food; and if remedial measures are to be taken it is essential to know the food sources of these nutrients, both for individuals and groups of people. With this information it is sometimes possible to explain clinical signs or laboratory findings in terms of omission or excess of individual foods or groups of foods in the diet. For example, it is known (DHSS 1972; 1975) that milk is, in the UK diet, the greatest single contributor of riboflavin. The finding that clinical signs of riboflavin deficiency and a low blood concentration of riboflavin correspond with low consumption of milk offers an immediate treatment – advice to increase milk consumption or, if this is not acceptable, alternative food sources of riboflavin or supplementation of the diet. Conversely, a knowledge of small intakes of milk, even in the absence of corroborative clinical evidence, can alert the physician to the possibility of future riboflavin deficiency. As yet there are relatively few data showing such clear causal relationships between individual foods and nutritional deficiencies, but further analysis of existing data and future work may provide information which could be the basis of a screening method for detecting individuals and groups who may be at risk.

INTERPRETATION OF FINDINGS
Explanation of dietary findings depends largely on a knowledge of the factors influencing the quantity and quality of food consumed, the availability to the individual who eats it of the nutrient content of this food and a knowledge of the physiological requirements of that individual.

No one has an absolutely free choice of food. Some foods are simply not obtainable, some are prohibitively expensive. Even when money and availability are not limiting factors choice can be affected in many ways. In old age some probable explanations of restricted diets are: poor appetite; apathy; restricted income; loneliness and bereavement; restricted mobility; mental status; poor dentition; and diseases resulting in malabsorption.

Dietary evidence needs to be related to these (and perhaps other) medical and social states if preventive and remedial measures are to be taken. The use of a computer is essential to analyse dietary data when appreciable numbers of subjects are surveyed and a large number of nutrients are to be calculated. The computer makes possible the use of sophisticated statistical methods. Discriminant analysis and multiple regression analysis will demonstrate correlations where they exist. Such correlations are not necessarily conclusive. A biological relationship may exist in the absence of a mathematical correlation and the reverse is equally true. Nevertheless, statistical analysis can indicate areas for further investigation, even when the biological association is not clear. The relative imprecision of the figures describing energy and nutrient intakes must be taken into account as must the fact that the typicality of the dietary data collected is presumed, not proven. If quicker, less expensive methods of conducting reliable dietary surveys are developed they will owe much to statistical analyses of existing and future data which may identify probable indices of the quality of a diet.

CONCLUSION

The purpose of nutrition studies of the elderly is threefold:

1. To discover the eating patterns and nutritional status of the elderly population selected.

2. To discover changes in eating pattern and nutritional status over a period of time and to explain such changes.

3. To throw some light on the question 'what is normal old age?' Health in old age appears to range from mental and physical infirmity at a relatively young age to an 'elite' group who, at a very advanced age, are healthy, active and alert.

The answer to the last question, if it can be found, has important personal, economic and social implications. Nutrition surveys, with all the limitations of the method of collecting and interpreting dietary data, have over the past 20 years contributed much knowledge and raised many questions. Much work remains to be done and more longitudinal studies are necessary, but progress to date is promising.

REFERENCES

Burke B. S. (1947) *J. Am. Diet. Assoc.* **23**, 1041.
Caird F. I., Judge T. G. and MacLeod C. (1975) *Gerontol. Clin. (Basel)* **17**, 47.
Davidson C. S., Livermore J., Anderson P. et al. (1962) *Am. J. Clin. Nutr.* **10**, 181.
Debry G., Bleyer R. and Martin J. M. (1977) *J. Hum. Nutr.* **31**, 195.
DHSS (1972) 3 (*see* General References).
DHSS (1975) *A Nutrition Survey of Pre-school Children.* 1967–68. Report on Health Social Subjects No. 10. London, HMSO.
Disselduff M. M. (1973) In: Howard A. N. and McLean Baird I. (ed.), *Nutritional Deficiencies in Modern Society.* London, Newman, p. 98.
Durnin J. V. G. A. and Blake E. C. (1962) *Br. J. Nutr.* **16**, 261.
Exton-Smith A. N. and Stanton B. R. (1965) KEHFa. (*see* General References).
Judge T. G., Caird F. I., Leask R. G. S. et al. (1974) *Age Ageing* **3**, 167.
Lonergan M. E., Milne J. S., Maule M. M. et al. (1975) *Br. J. Nutr.* **34**, 517.
MacLeod C. C. (1972) *Methods of Dietary Assessment.* Reprint from Symposia of the Swedish Nutrition Foundation X. 118.
Marr J. W. (1971) *World Rev. Nutr. Diet.* **13**, 105.
Steen B. (1977) In: *Nutrition in 70-year-olds. Dietary Habits and Body Composition. A report from the population study '70-year-old People in Gothenburg, Sweden'.* From the Department of Geriatric and Long-term Care Medicine and the Department of Clinical Nutrition, Sweden, University of Gothenburg.
Widdowson E. M. and McCance R. A. (1943) *Lancet* **1**, 230.
Wiehl D. G. (1942) *Milbank Mem. Fund. Q.* **20**, 329.
Young C. M. and Trulson M. F. (1960) *Am. J. Publ. Health* **50**, 803.

7. NUTRITIONAL STATUS: DIAGNOSIS AND PREVENTION OF MALNUTRITION
A. N. Exton-Smith

The dietary pattern in the majority of the elderly remains similar to that established by habits at a younger age, and their nutritional status continues to be adequate even in extreme old age. There are, however, many factors which begin to operate more frequently with increasing age and these may lead to nutritional deficiencies. They are due both to the changes in economic circumstances and way of life which often occur on retirement and to the increasing incidence of disease and disabilities which lead to alterations in dietary intake, absorption and metabolism of nutrients, occurring particularly during the eighth decade. In some instances there is an exaggeration in old age of faulty food habits which have been developed during earlier years.

RECOMMENDED INTAKES OF NUTRIENTS
Many countries have formulated 'standards' for energy and nutrient intakes and the recommendations for the United Kingdom have been published by the Department of Health and Social Security (1969). The values for elderly people are shown in *Table* 7.1.

The values given for energy requirements are similar to those recommended by the WHO/FAO (1973), except the UK values for elderly women are considerably higher. The recommendations for the elderly, however, are based on estimates of the average rate at which activities decline; that is, they take account of the diminution in energy expenditure associated with the increasing incidence of physical infirmity with age. Nevertheless, there are many individuals especially in rural communities whose activities are well maintained in old age and whose calorie intakes are much greater than the recommended values.

NUTRITIONAL STATUS
Most of our knowledge of the nutrition of the elderly population has been gained from cross-sectional surveys. Age differences have been established by the comparison of the results of measurements made on individuals of various age groups. These surveys have usually revealed that a proportion of subjects have low intakes of certain nutrients. In order to assess the effects on health of these low intakes serial investigations on the same

Table 7.1. Recommended daily intakes of energy and nutrients for elderly people in the UK (from DHSS, 1969)

	Men		Women	
	65–74	75+	55–74	75+
Energy (cal)	2350	2100	2050	1900
(MJ)	9·8	8·8	8·6	8·0
Protein (g)	59	53	51	48
Calcium (mg)	500	500	500	500
Iron (mg)	10	10	10	10
Thiamine (mg)	0·9	0·8	0·8	0·7
Riboflavine (mg)	1·7	1·7	1·3	1·3
Nicotinic acid (mg)	18	18	15	15
Ascorbic acid (mg)	30	30	30	30
Vitamin A (µg retinol equiv.)	750	750	750	750
Vitamin D (µg cholecalciferol)	2·5	2·5	2·5	2·5

individual are required. Moreover such longitudinal studies are the only means of clearly identifying the changes which are due to ageing. Ideally the repeated measurements (which must include dietary intake, medical examination and laboratory investigations) should be made on the same person at standardized intervals of time over as long a period as possible; for obvious reasons there have been few studies of this kind.

Cross-sectional Studies
There have been a number of nutritional surveys of random samples of old people at home and of the aged in residential homes. In a survey sponsored

Table 7.2. Mean daily intakes of calories and nutrients for women in the eighth decade

Calories	1890	Calcium (mg)	860
Protein (g)	57	Iron (mg)	9·9
Fat (g)	74	Vitamin C (mg)	37
Carbohydrate (g)	221	Vitamin D (iu)	135

by the King Edward's Hospital Fund for London (Exton-Smith and Stanton, 1965) an investigation was made of the diets of old people living alone at home in two North London Boroughs. The participants were 60 women whose ages ranged from 70 to 80 years (with the exception of three aged 89, 90 and 94 years). The mean daily intakes of nutrients were satisfactory and are shown in *Table* 7.2.

Few instances of malnutrition were revealed by the survey, but a proportion of the subjects had intakes of nutrients which were less than the recommended allowances, especially for iron and vitamin C. There was a striking correlation between diet and health; nearly all the subjects whose diet was better than average were judged on clinical assessment to be better than average in health. Although a good diet is undoubtedly one of the factors responsible for good health it is probably more likely that better health and greater physical activity are associated with good appetite and a larger intake of food.

When the 60 subjects were arranged in groups according to their ages a striking decrease in intakes of all nutrients with advancing age was found. *Table* 7.3 shows the percentage fall in mean intake for subjects in their late seventies compared with those in their early seventies.

Table 7.3. Cross-sectional study: fall in mean intake of nutrients during the eighth decade

Calories and nutrients	Fall in intake %
Calories	19
Protein	24
Fat	30
Carbohydrate	8
Calcium	18
Iron	29
Vitamin C	31

The age differences in intake revealed by this cross-sectional study might be the result of several factors:

1. Reduction in basal metabolic rate and lean body mass leading to a fall in physiological requirements with advancing age. Thus the decrease in intake may represent true age changes affecting all individuals.

2. A reduction in appetite and energy expenditure in some of the older subjects due to the development of disease or disability as they enter the second half of the eighth decade. It is known that there is a striking increase in the prevalence of incapacity in the elderly population after the age of 75 (Sheldon, 1948).

3. Individuals with dietary habits of excessive eating over many years may fail to reach extreme old age. Thus the dietary intake of the thinner individuals of the late 70's group would be expected to be less.

4. Secular differences between the two groups in that the lifelong dietary pattern of the older group may have been different from that of the early seventies group. Indeed it is possible that the habitual dietary pattern may have been one of the factors responsible for the longevity of those who reach extreme old age.

This cross-sectional study must be interpreted as revealing interesting age differences between the two groups and it was not possible to determine the relative importance of the four factors. The most important, however, was believed to be the influence of disease and disability affecting particularly the older subjects. Further evidence that low intakes of nutrients are associated with impairment of health in old age was obtained from a study of the nutrition of housebound elderly people (Exton-Smith et al., 1972). The intakes of the housebound were compared with age-matched active people, and for women the differences amounted to 15 per cent less for carbohydrate to 46 per cent less for vitamin C. For the housebound group as a whole there was no decline in intake with advancing age. This is because for the housebound, in contrast with the active group, disability was just as severe in the younger as in the older people. It can be concluded that disability has a greater influence on nutrient intake than the effects of increasing age alone.

Longitudinal Studies
The 60 women who participated in the first King Edward's Hospital Fund survey were followed up to form a longitudinal study and the 22 women who were still alive and could be traced were re-examined six-and-a-half years later (Stanton and Exton-Smith, 1970). It was found that for those subjects who maintained their health (as assessed on clinical examination and by a scoring system recording physical disabilities) the intakes of nutrients in the two surveys were remarkably similar. But for those women whose health had declined there was considerable fall in intake amounting on average to 20 per cent for protein and 17 per cent for calories. From this limited study it was confirmed that nutrient intakes in old age are usually maintained provided the person remains active and fit, and that physical disability is the most likely cause of declining intakes in the elderly.

One of the first longitudinal studies designed to assess the nutritional status of the elderly was carried out in San Mateo, California. The initial survey on 577 subjects over the age of 50 was conducted in 1948—49 and all but 47 patients lived in their own homes (Gillum and Morgan, 1955). When the data from the first survey were analysed on a cross-sectional basis by comparing the nutrient intakes of subjects in the three age groups, 55—64, 65—74, and 75 years and over it was found that there was a progressive fall in intakes with age, especially after the age of 75 years. These results were similar to those found in the first survey of the King Edward's Hospital Fund. Further studies were conducted 4, 6, and 14 years later (Chope and Breslow, 1956; Steinkamp et al., 1965) and there were 141 participants in all four surveys. Although a reduction in intake after the age of 75 occurred there was no significant difference between the four studies in the proportion of calories contributed by carbohydrate, protein and fat, for any of the groups. Moreover, there was little alteration with age in individual intakes of animal protein; those subjects with low intakes in 1948 tended to maintain the same pattern through to 1962. When interpreting these results it is still not possible to determine whether the life-long nutritional pattern of those who reach extreme old age has contributed to their longevity or whether their heredity which has enabled them to survive has also in some manner characterized their nutrition (Watkin, 1968).

MALNUTRITION

Malnutrition may be defined as a disturbance of form or function due to lack of (or excess of) calories or of one or more nutrients (DHSS, 1972). This definition includes both obesity and undernutrition. Obesity is a problem in old age and after the age of 75 it is much more common in women than in men, but it usually results from longstanding faulty eating habits. Undernutrition, on the other hand, results from environmental and physical factors which usually affect people in later life.

Causes

From the point of view of prevention of malnutrition it is of practical value to consider the causes of malnutrition under two headings; namely, social and environmental factors, and physical and mental disorders affecting the individual. The adverse social and environmental factors include ignorance, poverty and unfavourable domestic circumstances, especially those associated with social isolation and loneliness, lack of help in the home and inadequate cooking facilities. These factors are often associated with other unmet social needs so that malnutrition due to these causes does not occur in isolation. The internal disorders, both physical and mental that can lead to malnutrition include impaired appetite associated with constitutional diseases, masticatory inefficiency, physical disabilities, mental disturbances (depression as well as dementia) malabsorption and partial gastrectomy, alcoholism and the effect of drugs, and in some cases an increased requirement for nutrients. The environmental factors can often be alleviated by improved public health measures, whereas the internal conditions may or may not respond to appropriate medical treatment.

1. Adverse Social and Environmental Factors

a. Ignorance. The King Edward's Hospital Fund survey (Exton-Smith and Stanton, 1965) showed that ignorance of the basic facts of nutrition is prevalent in elderly women. Their views had often been formulated many years ago, even in childhood, when dietary habits had been dictated by financial stringency. It is likely that in men ignorance is even more important, especially in certain sections of the elderly population. Thus a man who is recently widowed may have to fend for himself for the first time and he may have little idea of what constitutes a balanced diet. Widower's scurvy is seen most often in the man living alone and eating mostly packaged food, tea, bread, butter and jam.

b. Poverty. The food eaten by pensioners is often dull, monotonous and tasteless. Brockington and Lempert (1967) in the Stockport survey of the social needs of the over 80s, showed that old people who are able to supplement their income from savings or from part-time earnings have a better diet than those whose sole financial means is the old age pension. In the winter months many old people must make a choice between spending money on food or fuel. Thus poverty is a factor to be considered in the elderly more often than in other age groups.

c. Social Isolation. Brockington and Lempert (1967) showed that dietary intake was related to the number of outside interests of old people. Dietary intake was found to be better in those old people who eat at clubs in the company of others. By contrast for many old people living alone in social isolation there is loss of interest sometimes amounting to apathy and consequent neglect in the preparation of food. What food is eaten is usually taken in the form of snacks.

Malnutrition also occurs in this group which includes old people suffering from chronic brain syndrome and confusional states. Perhaps even more important is the association between malnutrition and depressive illness, which leads to a disinclination to obtain, to cook and, even in severe cases, to eat food.

2. Internal Disorders

a. Malabsorption. Mild degrees of malabsorption are not uncommon in the elderly. This may be due to small bowel ischaemia, gluten sensitivity and other causes. The absorption of fat and fat-soluble vitamins and of folic acid and vitamin B_{12} is mainly affected. The sequelae of partial gastrectomy include protein—calorie malnutrition, anaemia due to iron, folate and vitamin B_{12} deficiency, and osteomalacia due to vitamin D deficiency.

b. Alcohol and Drugs. When alcohol intake is excessive, calorie needs may be derived mainly from this source and the intake of other nutrients may be curtailed. Folic acid metabolism is impaired in some alcoholics and megaloblastic anaemia can occur: it is also impaired in those taking barbiturates and anticonvulsant drugs and in those receiving cytotoxic agents, such as methotrexate. Enzyme induction by anticonvulsant drugs can also lead to vitamin D deficiency.

c. Increased Requirements. Negative nitrogen balance and the breakdown of tissue protein can occur in patients who are immobilized in bed for long periods, in those who suffer from long-continued pyrexia and as a result of extensive bedsores with the loss of protein-rich fluid. The extent to which this can be reversed by high supplemental intakes of protein is uncertain.

Vulnerable Groups

Often several of the various factors described operate together to produce malnutrition in the individual. Sometimes the combining factors are inter-related; for example, limited mobility, loneliness, social isolation and depression are all found in housebound old people and make them especially liable to malnutrition when they are receiving insufficient support from others.

Sheldon (1948), in a survey of a random sample of the elderly population of Wolverhampton, investigated the capacity for movement of old people. He found that 2·5 per cent were bedfast and a further 8·5 per cent had limitation of movement which restricted them to the house. There was a striking increase in disability with age: for the age group 60—64 years 1·5 per cent were housebound, but for those aged 85 and over no less than 32 per cent were confined to the house. Sheldon demonstrated a clear relationship between loneliness and capacity for movement. The bedfast were the least lonely since they had constant human contacts derived from the need for nursing attention which had to be supplied in order to maintain them in their homes. On the other hand, the highest incidence of loneliness was found in those whose activities confined them to the house and it exceeded that found in the sample as a whole. Sheldon thought this was due to the fact that many of the subjects were well enough to be left alone at home all day but they were incapable of sufficient physical activity to keep them fully occupied.

The housebound have been found to have nutrient intakes which are substantially lower than those of active people matched for age (Exton-Smith et al., 1972). Since about 8 per cent of the elderly population are housebound, that is, about three-quarters of a million people in Great Britain, this section of the population represents the largest single group vulnerable to malnutrition. Thus disability in old age not only affects the mode of living of those afflicted but it also has an adverse effect on dietary intakes and nutritional status.

Incidence

The results of the 'Nutrition Survey of the Elderly' (DHSS, 1972) based on random samples of old people living at home in six areas of the United Kingdom show that malnutrition occurs in about 3 per cent of the elderly population. This includes protein—calorie malnutrition, iron deficiency and several vitamin deficiencies. In the majority of cases it was a direct or indirect consequence of physical or mental disorder. Nevertheless, primary causes related to mode of living and other socio-economic factors may be of importance. Thus in the absence of overt malnutrition it was found that men over the age of 75 living alone fared worse than those living with a relative or spouse in respect of a large number of nutrients, and this was in some measure reflected in the proportion having biochemical levels below certain arbitrary limits; for example, four times as many men over 75 years of age living alone had leucocyte ascorbic acid levels below 7 $\mu g/10^8$ w.b.c. compared with those living in the company of others. Similarly, both for men and women, there was a statistically significant higher incidence of anaemia in those living alone compared with that found in other groups.

Detection of Malnutrition

The clinical significance of malnutrition is far greater than its incidence might suggest, since in almost every case it is treatable with excellent results. Difficulties in detection of the early signs of malnutrition are similar to those encountered in the early recognition of many diseases in old age. But in the case of nutritional deficiencies there are two further difficulties: for almost every nutrient there is a long latent period before a low intake leads to overt clinical manifestations and early diagnosis must depend upon the findings of abnormalities in special tests, including biochemical and haematological investigations; secondly, in the elderly the true significance of departures from normality revealed by these tests is unknown. Many of the abnormalities can be related to low intakes of certain nutrients, but in old age there is considerable variation between individuals. In general, it should be remembered that in younger persons the margin of safety is wide, but in old age homeostatic mechanisms are often impaired and the precarious physiological balance may be upset by the operation of medical and environmental hazards to which the elderly are prone. Frank malnutrition may be precipitated by such stress in those individuals whose nutrition is only marginally adequate (Exton-Smith, 1968).

PREVENTION OF MALNUTRITION

The salient features of the nutritional deficiencies which are revealed by population surveys and which are relevant to the problem of the prevention of malnutrition in the elderly can be summarized as follows:

1. A significant proportion of older people have low dietary intakes and many of these are well below the recommended nutrient intakes for the United Kingdom. In some instances there is an association between low intakes and socio-economic factors (for example, living alone) and with physical disorders, especially those which render the individual housebound.

2. Many old people have blood and tissue levels of nutrients that are below the arbitrarily defined limits adopted for younger people. The lowest levels are often found in those individuals with physical disorders.

3. Only rarely are the low intakes and abnormal biochemical findings associated with a disturbance of form or function that is required for the diagnosis of clinical malnutrition.

4. The significance of subclinical malnutrition and the extent to which the health of these old people would benefit from increased dietary intakes are unknown. Nevertheless it would seem prudent to attempt to

raise the levels of nutrients in order to make these individuals more resistant to the effects of stress due to non-nutritional diseases which become increasingly common with advancing years.

In most forms of nutritional deficiency in the elderly the factors responsible can be identified. Malnutrition can occur in isolation but it is more often associated with other unmet medical and social needs. Thus a prime consideration in improving nutrition is the early ascertainment and correction of needs in vulnerable groups of the elderly population.

Identification of At-risk Factors

Old people especially at risk are the socially isolated; those with physical disability including impairment of the special senses which contribute to isolation; the recently bereaved; very old men living alone; and those with mental disorders, particularly depression. Unless these vulnerable groups can be identified preventive measures would have to be applied to all old people irrespective of the fact that the majority will never suffer from malnutrition. The undesirability and the inefficiency of applying such procedures can be overcome only by the recognition of those especially at risk. The application of preventive measures to these smaller groups rather than to the entire elderly population then becomes a manageable proposition.

The housebound, who account for nearly 8 per cent of old people living in their homes, constitute the largest group at risk. Physical and mental disorder in old age not only affects the mode of living and social relationships of those afflicted, but also the dietary pattern and nutritional status. Since the majority of the housebound are already known to the health and social services, the prevention of malnutrition in this group should present less difficulty than in other vulnerable groups who are not so readily identifiable.

Assessment of Nutritional Status

When the groups of old people especially at risk have been identified the prevention of malnutrition is the responsibility of the primary medical care team. Although the assessment of dietary intakes should ideally be made by dietitians, their skills are not often available for old people at home. A rough guide to the quality of the diet can be obtained by health visitors using simple scoring systems (for example, the method designed by Marr et al., 1961) which are based on the number of main meals and the frequency of consumption of certain foods containing protein (meat, bread, eggs, cheese and milk). If the diet is found to be insufficient means must be sought for improving nutritional intake; this may entail instruction by a dietitian or health visitor, either individually or when old people attend clubs or day centres. When clinical malnutrition is suspected the diagnosis can sometimes be confirmed by the general practitioner using appropriate biochemical and haematological investigations; in other instances, however, referral to hospital for more specialized investigations will be necessary, for example, for bone biopsy when there are clinical findings suggestive of osteomalacia.

Club Meals and Meals-on-Wheels

It has been shown that there is often an improvement in nutrient intake when old people eat at clubs in the company of others. Many find that it is more convenient to have a club meal since there is no shopping, cooking or washing-up to be done. The King Edward's Hospital Fund Survey (Exton-Smith and Stanton, 1965) showed that in order to make an effective contribution to the total dietary intake at least four club meals a week should be eaten. The club or domiciliary meal must be as nutritious as possible since the recipient tends to regard it as the main meal of the day and often takes only snacks at other times.

About 1·5 per cent of old people receive meals-on-wheels (DHSS, 1970) but the real need is probably much greater than this. The meals service is usually provided by the WRVS and the regular visits to the homes of housebound old people do much to prevent social isolation. One of the disadvantages of the present system of delivery is that food must be kept hot for several hours after cooking before the meal reaches the old person's home. During this period at least some of the nutritive value is lost. There is need for experiment in this field. In several areas the provision of frozen meals has been tried. The meal can be cooked immediately before it is eaten and since food is delivered only once a week the service is economical in personnel. The main disadvantages, however, are that there may be no proper facilities for cold storage, the patient may be unable to cook the meal himself and he is visited much less frequently by voluntary workers.

Nutrient Supplementation

The most satisfactory means of promoting good nutrition is by improving the quality, and in some cases the quantity, of the diet. Thus for those whose consumption of vitamin C is inadequate, intake could be improved by the addition of oranges, blackcurrant juice, rose hip syrup or tomatoes. The alternative of prescribing ascorbic acid tablets is satisfactory, but less desirable. The very low intake of vitamin D by many old people must lead to consideration of supplementation especially for the housebound. A means of increasing the intake would be by the fortification of milk, which is a procedure adopted in the United States.

It is important that supplementation should only be introduced after the results of carefully controlled trials are available to assess the benefits derived from increased intakes. Once the practice of supplementation has become widespread it becomes difficult to prove the benefits. Moreover, there is an understandable reluctance to withdraw a prophylactic measure on the basis of doubts about its value when it has been employed for several years.

REFERENCES

Brockington F. and Lempert S. M. (1976) *The Stockport Survey. The Social Needs of the Over 80's.* Manchester University Press.

Chope H. D. and Breslow L. (1956) *Am. J. Publ. Health* **46**, 51.

DHSS (1969) 120 (*see* General References).

DHSS (1970) 123 (*see* General References).

DHSS (1972) 3 (*see* General References).

Exton-Smith A. N. (1968) In: Exton-Smith and Scott (*see* General References).

Exton-Smith A. N. and Stanton B. R. (1965) KEHFa (*see* General References).

Exton-Smith A. N., Stanton B. R. and Windsor A. C. M. (1972) KEHFb (*see* General References).

Gillum H. L. and Morgan A. F. (1955) *J. Nutr.* **55**, 265.

Marr J. W., Heady J. A. and Morris J. (1961) In: *Proc. Third International Congress of Dietetics.* London, Newman.

Sheldon J. H. (1948) *The Social Medicine of Old Age.* London, Oxford University Press.

Stanton B. R. and Exton-Smith A. N. (1970) *A Longitudinal Study of the Dietary of Elderly Women.* London, King Edward's Hospital Fund.

Steinkamp R. C., Cohen N. L. and Walsh H. E. (1965) *J. Am. Diet. Assoc.* **46**, 103.

Watkin D. M. (1968) In: Exton-Smith and Scott (*see* General References).

WHO/FAO (1973) (*see* General References).

8. OBESITY
J. Runcie

Obesity is the commonest nutritional disorder of the developed countries (Mérimée, 1971). In the absence of a proper pathophysiological definition of obesity an obese subject is arbitrarily defined as any individual who exceeds his or her ideal weight by more than 10 per cent. Ideal weights are based on pooled American life assurance data relating age at death to body weight. These statistics underline the major hazard of obesity, premature death (Society of Actuaries, 1959). The maximum incidence of obesity is in middle adult life. Females, particularly the ageing parous subject, are more frequently affected than males.

Obesity is due to an abnormal accumulation of adipose tissue (fat) within the body resulting in a variable increase in body weight, its major physical characteristic. Throughout adult life in normal weight subjects a precise balance is achieved between food (energy) ingestion and energy expenditure. In obese subjects this balance is disturbed for reasons which are not yet apparent. Recent studies have shown that reduced physical activity rather than excessive food intake is the major functional abnormality in obese subjects (Johnson et al., 1956; Runcie and Hilditch, 1974).

Obesity in the aged has several distinguishing characteristics. The most obvious is the sex difference. Obesity, particularly severe obesity, is almost confined to the female. Male sex and obesity are not compatible with prolonged survival due to accelerated hypertension and degenerative vascular disease. Obesity rarely arises *de novo* in the elderly and hence aged obese subjects will reflect those factors which promote chronicity and therapeutic failure. A high incidence of complications, particularly osteoarthritis of the weight-bearing joints and non-insulin dependent diabetes mellitus, is seen in this group.

DIAGNOSIS AND MEASUREMENT

The usual, and until recently the only method of establishing a diagnosis of obesity, was by measurement of body weight. The severity of obesity can then be ascertained by reference to standard weight tables. This is valid provided that excess weight in the individual is not a consequence of an hypertrophied muscle mass, as may occur in some athletes. This latter is not associated with the metabolic abnormalities of established obesity

(Kalkhoff and Ferrou, 1971) and is unlikely to be encountered in the aged.

Obesity would be precisely defined if accurate techniques were available to measure body composition, i.e. the relative proportions of adipose tissue (fat) and lean tissue (muscle) in the body. Until recently body composition measurement was not possible. Anthropometric techniques have now been developed in an attempt to overcome this problem. These depend on measurements of skin fold thickness at defined sites in the body (mid-biceps, subscapular area) and by applying the relevant regression equations an estimate of total body fat content can be obtained (Durnin and Rahaman, 1967). Body density measurements obtained from weighing subjects in air and in water can be used similarly to estimate body fat content. These physical methods are however lacking in precision and so are of limited use for the individual obese subject.

Body composition and short term changes therein are best measured by a scanning type of whole-body monitor employing a ring of sodium iodide detectors, five usually, through which the patient is slowly passed to measure the naturally occurring isotope, ^{42}K. This provides a measurement of whole-body potassium in grams which is converted to kg lean body tissue. The method is accurate, non-invasive and ideally suited to investigative studies in patient groups such as the elderly. An extension of this principle is the recent description of whole-body nitrogen measurements using cyclotron excitation of the nitrogen nuclei to measure changes in lean tissue mass (Walsh et al., 1976). Since body weight is made up of two variable components, lean tissue and adipose tissue, and a relatively constant component, skeletal mass, serial measurements of these variables when (whole) body weight is changing will provide important data on the factors promoting, in this instance, lipogenesis.

NOVEL CLINICAL ASPECTS OF OBESITY IN THE AGED

A number of distinctive clinical facets of obesity may only be observed in the elderly, either because of the time interval required for their development or because the ageing process directly affects the development of obesity or promotes its complications.

Locomotor Disability

Osteoarthritis of the major weight-bearing joints (hips, knees) is an inevitable accompaniment of long-standing obesity. This has several effects. Mobility, already impaired, is restricted further. Energy expenditure is reduced and the disease is exacerbated. Chronic pain may lead to chronic analgesic ingestion which can result in significant gastrointestinal blood loss and the development of iron-deficiency anaemia. In a small number of subjects, prolonged analgesic consumption will cause renal disease — analgesic nephropathy — and increasing renal failure, which form is further complicated by secondary renal tubular acidosis. Impaired mobility has other untoward effects on the aged. The individual may become house-bound. The consequent failure to undergo ultraviolet exposure leads to vitamin D deficiency and metabolic bone disease. Limb pain in these circumstances may become so acute that weight bearing becomes impossible. Painful, subcutaneous fatty tissue (panniculitis) appears to be a particular problem in the elderly and in some patients this has been observed as the presenting and dominating complaint.

Hypothyroidism
The incidence of hypothyroidism increases with age and is a particular problem in the elderly. The fall in basal metabolism and diminution in physical activity seen here promotes obesity. A specific biochemical abnormality is to be observed, namely the failure of normally circulating catecholamines to promote lipolysis from adipose tissue in the absence of circulating thyroxine (Galton, 1971). The possibility of hypothyroidism complicating obesity should always be considered, particularly in the elderly female.

Diabetes Mellitus
Maturity onset diabetes mellitus is a major complication of obesity. It is a particular problem in the ageing obese female. Ageing *per se* is associated with an increase in the fasting blood glucose of some 7 mg per cent per decade of life (O'Sullivan, 1974).

Physical inactivity *per se*, a concomitant of obesity, causes glucose intolerance. The magnitude of this problem can be gauged from the fact that more than half of all newly diagnosed diabetics in middle and later life are obese and that diabetic eye involvement is the commonest cause of blindness in this age group in America (American Diabetes Association, 1976). In addition the elderly obese diabetic is more likely to suffer from peripheral neuropathy and the disabling problem of orthostatic hypotension from ischaemic involvement of the intermediolateral horn cells of the spinal cord. An excessive mortality from acute myocardial infarction has been reported in the obese diabetic female. This is a reversal of the normal outcome and merits further study (Tansey et al., 1977).

Miscellaneous Effects
Other particular problems of obesity in the elderly are the aggravation of intercurrent disease, the liability to vehicular accidents and the respiratory (ventilatory) failure that can develop in the massively obese with moderate obstructive airways disease which renders them somnolent and immobile — the Pickwick syndrome. The morbidity of obesity in the elderly is therefore greater than in the younger subject.

PSYCHOSOCIAL ASPECTS
To generalize, obesity is a product of female sex, multiparity and depressed socio-economic status. It is not only social-class related but is also

social-class mobile, i.e. an improvement in social status reduces the liability to obesity and vice versa. It is related to educational attainment and to the failure to develop a strong sense of self, a powerful body cathexis (Gold-blatt et al., 1965; Stunkard and Burt, 1967). Psychological studies have not demonstrated consistent abnormalities in obese subjects but anxiety has been encountered as a prominent neurotic feature in several studies (Silverstone, 1968).

The aetiological significance of these observations is not clear. A reasonable conceptual framework might be that obese subjects have a limited capacity to solve problems and when difficulties arise, e.g. marital, with children, in interpersonal relations, etc., chronic anxiety ensues and the individual retreats into solace eating and/or physical immobility. If this is correct it would be anticipated that the older subject would be less likely to be affected by such problems and would, through experience, have a greater capacity to resolve them. What little evidence there is regarding the outcome of treatment of obesity in the elderly could be interpreted as lending tenuous support to this hypothesis.

TREATMENT

The treatment of obesity is difficult (Stunkard and MacLaren-Hume, 1959). It has two separate components:

1. The promotion of weight loss, i.e. specific reduction in body adipose tissue.

2. The long-term maintenance of this reduced state.

Treatment will be considered under five headings: calorie restriction; drug therapy; starvation; surgical procedures; and psychotherapy.

Calorie Restriction

Reduction in food intake is the established therapy for obesity. This is based on a simple view of obesity as resulting from volitional over-eating by the obese subject, the severity and duration of caloric restriction being related to the severity of the obesity. This well-established but facile generalization has been, and continues to be, a major obstacle in the proper understanding of the obese process. The poor results of orthodox therapy (Stunkard and MacLaren-Hume, 1959) has resulted in a low patient expectation of success and has promoted an attitude of therapeutic nihilism in many physicians when confronted with this problem. It has failed to stimulate an interest into the almost uniquely intractable nature of inappropriate or non-physiological eating. It should be recognized that the obese subject is driven to eat by circumstances that are not appreciated and have been little considered. Reduction dieting should now be dis-carded from the therapeutic armamentarium as a significant therapy for established or severe obesity.

Drug Therapy

1. *Amphetamine*

The poor results of reduction dieting led to a search for appetite suppressing drugs as an adjunct to treatment. This led in turn to the introduction of amphetamine and its congeners into clinical practice, with unfortunate consequences. The drugs were stimulant to the nervous system, were addictive and in prolonged use were psychotomimetic. Weight reduction was at best transitory (Seaton et al., 1961). The use of such drugs in clinical practice for this purpose has been largely abandoned.

2. *Fenfluramine*

Attempts to dissociate the anorectic from the stimulant properties of amphetamine led to the development of a specific anorexiant drug, fenfluramine. Unfortunately its clinical use is attended by skin rashes, anorexia, sleep disturbance and withdrawal symptoms, whilst its clinical efficacy remains a matter of dispute.

3. *Bulk Agents*

The use of bulk agents such as methylcellulose to promote intestinal distension and hence satiety has attracted some interest but has failed to gain an established role in the management of obesity.

4. *Drug-induced Malabsorption*

Intestinal malabsorption is sometimes observed as an unwelcome drug side effect. The possibility of exploiting such effects in the therapy of obesity has been considered. Drugs known to cause malabsorption include neomycin and some sulphonamides. At present the possibility of causing permanent and irreparable damage to the small bowel mucosa limits their clinical use. They remain an interesting area for further study.

In addition to these specific drug therapies it is important to remember that the elderly are abnormally susceptible to drug toxicity for reasons that are not yet clearly defined; and, further, that the most serious toxic effects are to be encountered in this group (Hurwitz, 1969). At the present time, therefore, drug therapy has no established role to play in the treatment of obesity in the aged.

Starvation

Bloom (1959) reported that fasting (4–9 days) was well tolerated by obese subjects and that significant weight loss was achieved and maintained for periods in excess of nine months. Drenick et al. (1964) extended Bloom's original observations by showing that obese subjects could be fasted for periods much greater than had hitherto been considered physiologically possible (>100 days) and that massive weight loss could be achieved. They considered that patients with cardiac, hepatic and renal disease should not be fasted but gave no supportive evidence for these views. The studies of Thomson et al. (1966) and Runcie and Thomson (1970) further extended the scope of starvation. They demonstrated that the 'cure' of obesity, i.e. the attainment of a normal weight, by a single extended fast was possible. Prolonged starvation is attended by a small but definite risk of major complications; to date 5 deaths (4 female, 1 male) have been reported associated with this therapy.

1. *The Role of Starvation Therapy*

Starvation has an important role to play in the management of obesity in the aged, particularly in cases of massive or refractory obesity. It is in this group that obesity will most often be complicated by serious intercurrent disease – ischaemic heart disease, hypertension, diabetes mellitus and locomotor disorders – and in whom the related effects of starvation, e.g. a fall in the systemic blood pressure, an improvement in carbohydrate tolerance, in addition to weight loss, will have maximum therapeutic effect.

In practice the elderly obese subject tolerates extended starvation well, irrespective of the presence of intercurrent disease, with one proviso which will be discussed shortly. Weight loss is predictable. Proper patient monitoring (daily measurement of weight and urinary electrolyte excretion) will give ample warning of impending difficulties and allow appropriate corrective action to be taken. Finally the prolonged hospitalization which may be required presents less of a disruption to the older patient.

2. *Contraindication(s) to Therapeutic Starvation*

Three of the 5 reported deaths in fasting obese subjects have occurred in patients either in cardiac failure (1 death), or who had recently recovered from an episode of failure (2 deaths); a further death occurred in a young woman from ventricular fibrillation and cardiac standstill on re-feeding (Garnett et al., 1969). This has led practitioners of this therapy to adopt the clinical rule of thumb that no patient should undergo starvation therapy within a year of an episode of cardiac failure. This problem is most likely to be encountered in the aged.

A second, more theoretical problem occurs with obese subjects with hepatic disease. In the older person this is likely to be due to unsuspected chronic active liver disease. Overt hepatic disease is rarely complicated by obesity. Since the liver plays a central role in the metabolic response to starvation it is sensible to regard such subjects as unsuitable for this form of therapy.

3. *Modified, Protein-sparing Starvation*

Metabolic studies have shown that lean tissue breakdown continues throughout starvation. This effect is greatest initially (<14 days) and falls to a much reduced but constant level thereafter (Runcie and Hilditch,

1974). To maintain lean tissue mass the protein-sparing, modified fast was introduced in which carbohydrate-free, protein supplements (60–90 g/day) – formula diets – are given which allow net protein anabolism to continue (Lindner and Blackburn, 1976). Uncritical and poorly supervised use of these formula diets by obese subjects has been implicated in the deaths of 31 obese subjects in the United States (Center for Disease Control, quoted by Blackburn, 1978). In the hands of physicians experienced in the management of the obese and familiar with the pathophysiology of starvation this regimen has proved an effective therapy. The maintenance of protein homeostasis is a complex phenomenon, but a central requirement in conditions of protein–calorie deprivation. Humans are exquisitely adapted to privation, a phenomenon perhaps best demonstrated by the obese subject during extended starvation. The provision of protein supplements to fasting subjects may antagonize the complex metabolic adjustments to privation (starvation) and in that sense they may be contraindicated.

Surgical Treatment

There is much current interest in the surgical treatment of obesity. The now standard procedure is division of the jejunum and end-to-end anastomosis of its proximal end with the distal ileum, several inches above the ileocaecal valve. The adoption of such procedures underlines the intractable therapeutic problem of established and, in particular, massive obesity. There is a significant operative mortality (6 per cent); postoperative complications are frequent and include sudden death, intractable diarrhoea, oedema, phlebitis, renal calculi and recurrent electrolyte depletions and cirrhosis of the liver (Bray, 1977). The reported hazards of bypass surgery relate to the younger age groups (<50 years). Increasing age will exacerbate these problems. In the present state of knowledge, therefore, surgical bypass has little or no part to play in the management of obesity in the aged. Further it is difficult to believe that the complex psychosocial problems of the obese can be abolished by a stroke of the surgeon's knife.

Psychotherapy

The importance of psychotherapy in the obese depends on the physician's views of the aetiological significance of psychosocial events in this disorder. This is a controversial issue. Psychometric studies in the obese have not revealed a specific obese personality. It is undeniable that the obese population shows unusual but specific sex and social characteristics. Obesity is a disorder of the ageing, disadvantaged, parous female. Furthermore these characteristics are class-mobile, improvement in social grouping being associated with a lesser incidence of obesity and vice versa (Goldblatt et al., 1965). These group characteristics are well developed in the aged. A crucial problem in the management of obesity therefore becomes a knowledge and understanding of those factors which lead to the regaining of normal weight following pregnancy. From the admittedly fragmentary observations it is possible to construct a clinically useful model of the nature of obesity as follows: the obese subject has a traumatic or unacceptable life style. Long-standing inability to resolve difficulties (marital, emotional, etc.) promotes chronic anxiety. Relief from the latter is obtained by eating – the anxiolytic effect of food – and by retreating into physical inertia; but at the cost of increasing weight. This is consistent with the view that all behaviour is goal-orientated, i.e. the obese subject's inappropriate eating serves a more important purpose (for her) which is relief from anxiety. It is compatible with the observation of Simon (1963) that 'obesity is a depressive equivalent'. It suggests the reason that obesity may be so intractable therapeutically, requiring a major change in life style of the affected individual with all its attendant problems.

THE THERAPEUTIC PROGRAMME
Therapeutic Interview(s)
Obese subjects respond to sympathetic counselling. Feelings of guilt can be alleviated by a simple explanation of current views on the nature of obesity and why treatment failure is the rule rather than the exception. The origin of these obese subjects' obesity should be ascertained, an assessment of their personality made and a formal programme of weight loss instituted.

Weight Loss Programme
The weight loss programme will be dictated by the patient's clinical condition. In the massively obese, weight loss should be initiated by a period of supervised starvation in hospital for a minimum period of thirty days to achieve significant weight loss. Close outpatient follow-up is required on discharge. Monitoring of the domestic situation and elimination of poor or faulty eating habits can be achieved by home nursing visits, a facility being increasingly used in the management of the elderly.

Formal Psychotherapy
Patients will be encountered with major psychological difficulties. These should be fully dealt with in consultation with the psychologist and a programme of treatment, behaviour modification, group therapy etc. drawn up.

CONCLUSIONS
Obesity is a major health hazard in communities where food is readily and abundantly available. A major toll of the disease is exacted from aged obese subjects and seriously impairs the quality of life available to them. The failure of conventional therapy has led to a re-evaluation of the disease complex resulting in novel and effective forms of weight loss, which is not necessarily the same thing as cure of obesity; but in the

current climate of heightened research and clinical interest it is likely that resolution of this hitherto intractable problem can be achieved.

REFERENCES

American Diabetes Association (1976) *Fact Sheet on Diabetes.* New York, American Diabetes Assoc.

Blackburn G. L. (1978) *Obes. Bariatr. Med.* **7**, 25.

Bloom W. L. (1959) *Metabolism* **8**, 214.

Bray G. A. (1977) *Diabetes* **26**, 1072.

Drenick E. J., Swendsied M. E., Blahd W. H. et al. (1964) *J. Am. Med. Assoc.* **187**, 100.

Durnin J. V. G. A. and Rahaman M. M. (1967) *Br. J. Nutr.* **21**, 681.

Galton D. J. (1971) *The Human Adipose Cell.* London, Butterworths, p. 119.

Garnett E. S., Barnard D. L., Ford J. et al. (1969) *Lancet* **1**, 914.

Goldblatt P. B., Moore M. E. and Stunkard A. J. (1965) *J. Am. Med. Assoc.* **192**, 1039.

Hurwitz N. (1969) *Br. Med. J.* **1**, 536.

Johnson M. L., Burke B. S. and Mayer J. (1956) *Am. J. Clin. Nutr.* **4**, 37.

Kalkhoff R. and Ferrou C. (1971) *N. Engl. J. Med.* **284**, 1236.

Lindner P. G. and Blackburn G. L. (1976) *Obes. Bariatr. Med.* **5**, 198.

Mérimée T. J. (1971) *N. Engl. J. Med.* **285**, 856.

O'Sullivan J. B. (1974) *Diabetes* **23**, 713.

Runcie J. and Hilditch T. E. (1974) *Br. Med. J.* **2**, 352.

Runcie J. and Thomson T. J. (1970) *Br. Med. J.* **3**, 432.

Seaton D. A., Duncan L. J. P., Rose K. et al. (1961) *Br. Med. J.* **1**, 1009.

Silverstone J. T. (1968) *Proc. R. Soc. Med.* **112**, 371.

Simon R. I. (1963) *J. Am. Diet. Assoc.* **183**, 208.

Society of Actuaries (1959) Build and Blood Pressure Study.

Stunkard A. J. and Burt V. (1967) *Am. J. Psychol.* **123**, 1443.

Stunkard A. J. and MacLaren-Hume M. (1959) *Arch. Int. Med.* **103**, 79.

Tansey M. J. B., Kennelly B. M. and Opie L. H. (1977) *Br. Med. J.* **1**, 1624.

Thomson T. J., Runcie J. and Miller V. (1966) *Lancet* **2**, 992.

Walsh C. H., Soler N. G., James H. et al. (1976) *Q. J. Med.* **178**, 295.

9. GASTROINTESTINAL FUNCTION AND ABSORPTION OF NUTRIENTS
S. G. P. Webster

Deficiencies of nutrients may result from two different mechanisms in the gastrointestinal tract. First, functional impairment may lead to malabsorption and secondly, damaged areas may lead to nutrient loss. That is to say that the gut can be both the portal of entry of nutrients or the site of excessive loss. The relationship between nutrition and absorption is also a reciprocal arrangement: impairment of either will be detrimental to the other. The mucosal lining of the bowel, especially the small bowel, has one of the fastest rates of cell turnover in the body. This essential cell proliferation is a great consumer of nutrients, and as a consequence any dietary deficiency is likely to have an adverse effect on the health of the mucosa (Saraya et al., 1971). Both structure and function are significantly altered by deficiencies (Varito, 1962).

Tropical sprue (not a common problem in Western geriatric practice, but Price et al. (1977) describe 2 patients) clearly illustrates this close inter-relationship. Affected patients will suffer from severe folate deficiency, the correction of which is an important principle of treatment and helps in the restoration of normal small bowel function. Less dramatic, but of more relevance, is the demonstration of changes in the small bowel of patients with either vitamin B_{12} or folic acid deficiencies (Foroozan and Trier 1967; Bianchi et al., 1970). Falaiye (1971) has also demonstrated the correction of malabsorption after protein repletion in previously hypoproteinaemic subjects.

The interdependence of nutrition and absorption offers a fine example of one of the many vicious circles in medicine. The worsening of one factor leads to rapid acceleration and to complete failure (*Fig.* 9.1).

A fund of knowledge concerning nutritional problems in the elderly is now available and is well described in other chapters of this book. Unfortunately, the information concerning malabsorption in the last third of life is much more scanty. The high incidence of pathology in this age group makes the potential frequency of impaired absorption very high. The intestinal consequences, however, may be overshadowed by more dramatic changes in other systems. It is known that fairly gross pathological changes in the gastrointestinal tract may be very silent in old age (Cohen and Gitman, 1960).

The few studies which have been made have all been carried out on ill or disabled old people, either temporarily or permanently resident in an institution. From the work of Pelz et al. (1968), it would seem that at least 7 per cent of the residents of an old peoples' home showed some evidence of malabsorption or maldigestion. Twenty-three per cent of geriatric inpatients have been shown to have impaired xylose absorption (using a test which eliminates renal factors), 7 per cent at a level of severity found in younger patients with coeliac disease (Webster, 1973).

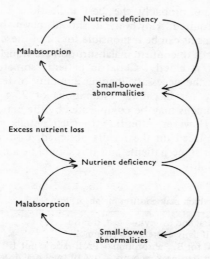

Fig. 9.1. The vicious cycles of deficiency and disease.

We remain ignorant of details of the absorptive functions of the 95 per cent of elderly people living in the community. The frequency of biochemical and haematological abnormalities which may be due to malabsorption should warn us of the potential extent of functional impairment.

When clinically significant malabsorption does occur in an elderly person, it is more likely to present via a complication than as a troublesome gut symptom. Even when excessive faecal fat excretion can be demonstrated, the patient is not usually aware of steatorrhoea. When the latter is obvious it is more likely to be due to maldigestion (usually pancreatic disease) than malabsorption. In fact, diarrhoea, apart from spurious diarrhoea secondary to faecal impaction, is a rare symptom in old age. When it does occur, an endocrine, infective or inflammatory cause needs to be sought.

The finding of a macrocytic anaemia, resistant iron-deficiency anaemia,

Table 9.1. Results which *may* indicate malabsorption

i.	Low serum iron
ii.	Low red cell folate
iii.	Low serum B_{12}
iv.	Hypoalbuminaemia
v.	Biochemical osteomalacia (low calcium and phosphorus, raised alkaline phosphatase)

or osteomalacia are probably the best indications that tests for mal-absorption are required. However, it should never be forgotten that alternative mechanisms can be responsible for all of these abnormalities.

The investigations to confirm malabsorption are fraught with difficulties when the subject is elderly. Geriatric patients sometimes find it very difficult to ingest the necessary loading amounts of test substances, e.g. 100 g of fat daily for faecal fat estimations or 25 g of d-xylose. The collection of specimens may be complicated by the patients' forgetfulness or incontinence. However, attention to such details is essential if any reliance is to be placed on the results obtained. Continuous supervision will be required of some patients and this should be a medical rather than a nursing responsibility.

Table 9.2. Tests which may confirm malabsorption

i.	Combined oral and i.v. xylose test, if ratio $<1{\cdot}8$
ii.	Faecal fats, if daily excretion >18 mmol
iii.	Dycopac test for B_{12} absorption – PA if ratio is not 1. Ileal defect if urinary recovery $<10\%$ of total oral dose – but of doubtful value in the elderly

Changes in other systems will invalidate the results of some tests. Impaired renal function is the greatest problem and effectively makes the standard Schilling Test (Rath et al., 1957) and d-xylose (Kendall, 1970) useless in old people. However, the combining of results from oral and intravenous xylose tests and the use of double isotopes and intrinsic factor (Katz et al., 1963) are methods of circumventing these problems. The necessary modifications of the xylose test are described by Kendall and Nutter (1970). The readily available Dycopac test is a useful method of examining B_{12} absorption in the elderly. Patients with pernicious anaemia are clearly identified: the remaining minority will have a defect in their terminal ileum or a structural abnormality in the small bowel, leading to abnormal bacterial colonization. A barium meal and follow-through will then be helpful in separating these final two groups.

Details of the methods used to establish the specific cause for mal-absorption will be given when each is discussed. It should be remembered that many will be due to gut involvement by a more widespread disorder. A full and complete history, past and present, and a careful general examination are therefore essential and may obviate the necessity of difficult and uncomfortable gastrointestinal investigation.

Table 9.3. Guidelines on how to investigate malabsorption

i.	Exclude malnutrition
ii.	Exclude maldigestion – usually pancreatic High faecal fat with normal xylose absorption Try effect of pancreatic extract on symptoms
iii.	Exclude generalized condition affecting gut
iv.	Folate deficiency with normal intake suggests small bowel disease, therefore do jejunal biopsy and combined xylose tests
v.	High folate plus low B_{12} suggests abnormal colonization, e.g. small bowel diverticular disease, therefore do barium meal and follow-through
vi.	Low B_{12} – either pernicious anaemia ⎫ or terminal ileal defect e.g. Crohn's ⎬ Do Dycopac test or stagnant loop or diverticulum ⎭ Do barium follow-through
vii.	Osteomalacia with folate deficiency – small bowel disease without folate deficiency – stagnant loop

Even the normal gut is a site of nutrient loss, e.g. iron in haemoglobin and small quantities of protein. Reabsorption of these substances usually keeps the loss at an insignificant level. However, impaired absorption will lead to decompensation, and damaged areas of gut act often as effective sites of excess loss.

Pathological processes, affecting parts of the gut not closely associated with absorption, may give rise to serious blood and serum loss leading to iron deficiency and hypoproteinaemia. The latter is usually nonselective, unlike renal protein loss, but hypoalbuminaemia is most obvious and troublesome. Excessive electrolyte loss is often associated with lesions in the large bowel.

The measurement of excess protein loss into the gut is extremely difficult and the results obtained are not always reliable. The problems become even greater in the elderly and it is often more realistic to exclude other causes of hypoproteinaemia (malnutrition, malabsorption, proteinuria and impaired synthesis) rather than make attempts to confirm excess loss into the gut.

THE STOMACH

The key to many gastric pathologies appears to be the presence of underlying chronic gastritis. This theory seems to apply to peptic ulceration, carcinoma and parietal cell malfunction.

Andrews et al. (1967) demonstrated a rising incidence of body gastritis with increasing age. There also appears to be an association between chronic gastritis and ulceration with atheroma (Elkeles, 1964; Jones et al., 1970). Achlorhydria becomes more common with increasing age and this is the first and most severe consequence of chronic gastritis.

Gastritis and iron deficiency often occur together, but it seems that the gastritis is responsible for the iron deficiency. Correction of the latter fails to improve the appearance of the gastric mucosa (Ikkala et al., 1970). Severe atrophic gastritis leads to increased gastric blood loss and protein secretion. Coghill (1969) has suggested that the protein loss may be sufficient to cause significant hypoproteinaemia.

Failure of intrinsic factor production closely follows the progressive reduction in acid secretion. The iron deficiency which may occur as a consequence of achlorhydria may be sufficient to precipitate pernicious anaemia in a patient previously capable of production of at least small amounts of intrinsic factor.

In the final stages of atrophic gastritis, the patient is likely to show iron deficiency due to gastric bleeding, hypoproteinaemia due to gastric protein loss and pernicious anaemia due to failure of intrinsic factor production. These patients are all at considerable risk of progressing to malignant change (Mosbech and Videbaek, 1950; Morson, 1955; Siurala and Seppala, 1960). Gastric carcinoma is also another recognized cause of protein-losing gastroenteropathy (Waldmann, 1970).

In patients who have undergone a partial gastrectomy, the risks of nutritional deficiencies are markedly increased. The gastric remnant is likely to show changes of gastritis (Stalsberg and Taksdal, 1971), and iron, B_{12} and protein deficiencies are common. In addition, malabsorption of other nutrients may arise as a result of the operation. The small bowel mucosa has been demonstrated to be abnormally flat in some post-gastrectomy patients (Joske and Blackwell, 1959; Scott et al., 1964) and carbohydrate and folic acid absorption is likely to be impaired in these patients. A further complication can be the development of steatorrhoea via the 'blind loop' mechanism. This may lead to malabsorption of fat-soluble vitamins. Clinically, vitamin D deficiency and subsequent osteomalacia is likely to be the most serious outcome. Chalmers (1968) described 38 patients (41 per cent of his series) who developed osteomalacia – the mean delay between operation and diagnosis was 11·4 years. Those patients who underwent gastric surgery late in life seemed to be at greatest risk.

It should also be remembered that all gastric pathologies are likely to be associated with loss of appetite. The combination of poor intake, poor absorption and excess nutrient loss are likely to summate to cause general debility and specific deficiencies.

DISORDERS OF THE SMALL BOWEL
Small bowel morphology is difficult to interpret in the elderly. Ageing itself is probably associated with the development of shorter and wider

jejunal villi (Webster and Leeming, 1975a, b). Abnormalities as gross as partial villous atrophy and subtotal villous atrophy were found amongst 5 per cent of geriatric patients with either biochemical or haematological evidence of malabsorption (Webster, 1973).

Coeliac Disease

This is sometimes diagnosed for the first time in patients over the age of 65 years. Badenoch (1960) describes 4 cases amongst 74 and Price et al. (1977) on investigating 47 patients above the age of 50 with steatorrhoea, found that 4 patients over 65 had coeliac disease which had not been previously diagnosed.

However, some doubt remains about the accuracy of the diagnosis, as the only sure test is a repeat jejunal biopsy after a trial with a gluten-free diet. The diagnosis is only confirmed if the mucosa has returned to normal on treatment.

Another dilemma is caused by the fact that a strict gluten-free diet is not justified in the elderly, unless it is the only way of controlling severe bowel symptoms. If properly adhered to, the diet is inconvenient; in young patients, the effort is repaid by the reduction in the risk of developing a small bowel neoplasm. Pathologies in other systems have a greater influence on prognosis in old patients, and the pleasures of a normal diet should not be denied the patient. Nutritional deficiencies can easily be corrected by supplementation: folic acid, vitamin D and iron are most likely to be required.

Jejunal Diverticulosis

This condition is more likely to occur in the elderly than in any other age group; cases are well described by Clark (1972). The diverticula act as blind or stagnant areas which are vulnerable to colonization by abnormal bacteria. The organisms may then interfere with fat absorption, and hence fat-soluble vitamins, by deconjugating bile salts. In addition, B_{12} may be consumed by the bacteria and blood loss may occur from the pouches if irritation and trauma take place. Nutritional problems likely to affect the patient are anaemia, due to either B_{12} or iron deficiency or both, and osteomalacia. The patient may also be troubled by intermittent diarrhoea or steatorrhoea.

If suspected, the diagnosis is most easily confirmed by performing a barium meal and follow-through in order to demonstrate the structural abnormalities. Extra diagnostic support may be obtained by estimating urinary indicans, which should be raised. The contents of the diverticula can be aspirated, but this causes considerable inconvenience to the patient and the culture techniques for the responsible organisms are difficult.

A therapeutic trial with a broad-spectrum antibiotic, usually tetracycline, is easily justified. It should be remembered that the lesions are always liable to recolonization and repeated courses of treatment may be required. If the diverticula are very extensive and troublesome they can be removed surgically.

Small Bowel Lymphoma

Although a rare cause of malabsorption it usually affects the elderly, and the lesions are most commonly of a diffuse and infiltrating type. Symptoms often include abdominal pain and mechanical complications such as obstruction, intussusception and perforation. The first clue to the diagnosis may be the demonstration of a malabsorption pattern on barium studies (Naqvi et al., 1969).

Patients with long-standing coeliac disease which has not been treated with a gluten-free diet are at risk from developing small bowel lymphomata (Gough et al., 1962).

The prognosis for both groups of patients is poor and treatment can only be of a supportive nature.

SYSTEMIC DISEASES AFFECTING THE GUT

Isolated attacks of acute conditions will sometimes have dramatic effects on the gut, but if the patient is normally healthy and makes a good recovery there will be no lasting effects on his nutritional state. It is therefore in chronic, slowly progressive disorders that we find evidence of nutritional impairment. In some cases this will simply be a reflection of financial and functional difficulties which accompany such chronic disorders and make a full and balanced diet impossible.

However, in a number of disorders there is evidence of direct involvement of the gut. A proportion of patients with scleroderma show signs of alimentary disorders: increased rigidity and immobility of the gut wall can easily be demonstrated on barium studies. The lack of mobility may enable bacteria to colonize parts of the lumen and absorption may be embarrassed (McBrien and Lockhart-Mummery, 1962).

Other conditions which primarily affect the skin – psoriasis and dermatitis herpetiformis are in addition, well recognized as having gut involvement (Marks and Shuster, 1968; Barry et al., 1971). Flattening of the small bowel mucosa can be as severe as that seen in coeliac disease. In these patients, the high cell turnover in both the dermis and jejunal mucosa helps to exacerbate the effects of malabsorption, and the converse is also true.

In rheumatoid arthritis, there is an increased need for nutrients because of the cellular proliferation in the synovial membranes. The described jejunal changes of flattening and broadening of the villi (Pettersson et al., 1970) may be due to folate deficiency. Alternatively, arterial changes could be responsible. Whatever the mechanism, impaired absorption is the likely result.

Degenerative arterial disease is undoubtedly one of the commonest pathologies which accompany ageing. Arterial narrowing adversely affects the function of the gut, just as it does the heart, kidney and brain. Abdominal angina has been recognized for many years. Its main symptom is central abdominal pain after meals (the larger the meal, the more severe the pain). Differentiation from other forms of dyspepsia, especially peptic ulceration, is difficult. Helpful clues, suggestive of an arterial aetiology, are aortic calcification and the presence of an abdominal bruit. The diagnosis can only be confirmed by arteriography, but this is rarely justified in the elderly, unless an isolated arterial lesion is suspected (Dick et al., 1967; Droller, 1972). In patients with widespread mesenteric ischaemia, severe deficiencies can occur: this is probably the result of poor nutrient intake, as food precipitates symptoms, plus impaired mucosal efficiency.

Milledge (1972) has demonstrated that patients with anoxia have impaired absorptive abilities. Severe congestive cardiac failure has the same effect (Hyde and Loehry, 1968), but venous congestion as well as anoxia may be adding a contribution. Clearly patients with chronic anoxia and venous congestion are liable to nutritional deficiencies – poor appetite, poor diet, continuous potent medication and impaired efficiency of the jejunal mucosa, all potentially occurring together.

A similar mixed aetiology is likely to be responsible for many of the deficiencies recorded in patients with malignant disease (Dymock et al., 1967).

HORMONES AND THE GUT

Diarrhoea is a well accepted feature of thyrotoxicosis and if severe will contribute to the wasting and dehydration seen in some patients. Thyroxine levels should certainly be checked in elderly patients with persistent diarrhoea or obscure weight loss.

Other diagnoses which need consideration in the same situation are those where hormones are produced by gut cells. These hormones will sometimes have distant as well as local actions.

Diarrhoea is frequently the presenting symptom of a carcinoid tumour, the flushing, wheezing and cardiac complications only occurring when liver metastases are present. A urinary estimation of 5-hydroxyindole acetic acid is required as the first step in confirming the diagnosis. If positive, barium studies will be required to locate the site of the lesion.

Another syndrome which presents with diarrhoea and is caused by hormone secreting alimentary tumours is that described by Zollinger and Ellison in 1955. Increased gastrin secretion is the responsible mechanism and a high serum level can be demonstrated (McGuigan and Trudeau, 1968). The function of pancreatic enzymes may be impaired by the resulting hyperacidity and maldigestion may follow. In addition, small bowel mucosal changes have been reported and malabsorption may occur (Summerskill, 1959). This disorder may be part of the pluriglandular syndrome and be associated with other endocrine disturbances.

In the Verner–Morrison syndrome, the presenting picture consists of severe watery diarrhoea combined with hypokalaemia and achlorhydria (Murray et al., 1961). It is a very rare clinical problem and results from hormone secretion (possibly secretin or gastrin and glucagon) by a non-beta islet cell tumour of the pancreas (Barbezat and Grossman, 1971).

DRUG-INDUCED DEFICIENCIES

There are four ways in which drugs may influence the availability and absorption of nutrients: appetite suppression; drug interactions; impairment of absorption; and excess loss of nutrients.

Appetite suppression may be a primary or secondary property of a drug. The primary suppressants such as diethylpropion hydrochloride (Tenuate) are not recommended for use in the elderly. Side-effects such as anxiety, agitation and cardiovascular complications are likely to be more troublesome than in younger patients. However, many drugs with clear indications for prolonged use in elderly patients may have an adverse effect on appetite. Spironolactone in the treatment of fluid retention is a common example. Many of the anti-inflammatory analgesics impair enjoyment and enthusiasm for food because of their dyspeptic side effects. Other drugs are more likely to be troublesome when taken in excessive doses. Digitalis preparations provide the best examples: the vomiting and weight loss seen in such patients may be sufficient to suggest a serious gastric pathology such as a carcinoma.

Oral iron and tetracycline if taken together chelate and both become unavailable for absorption.

Anticonvulsant therapy may lead to folate deficiency, several mechanisms being responsible. One depends on the effect of the drugs on conjugase activity in the small bowel mucosal cells (Rosenberg et al., 1969; Gerson et al., 1972). When the enzyme concentration is reduced, the main folate form in the diet, the polyglutamates, are not broken down, and the folate remains unavailable. This is one of the reasons why 75 per cent of epileptics on treatment have reduced serum folate levels and 38 per cent have a megaloblastic marrow (Reynolds et al., 1966).

Diabetics on long-term treatment with biguanides are also at risk of developing a macrocytic anaemia. In these cases, the deficiency is most likely to be of B_{12}, the absorption of which is impaired by the drugs (Stowers and Bewsher, 1969; Jounela et al., 1974). Other nutrients, including folate, can also be malabsorbed (Berchtold et al., 1971).

Alcohol has been shown to have a direct toxic effect on the small bowel mucosa, and this is one of the mechanisms of folate deficiency in alcoholics (Hermos et al., 1972) but a poor diet is frequently partly responsible.

Laxatives are used more frequently by the elderly than by any other group. If taken in excess, the resulting purging may lead to severe hypokalaemia. Patients who consume large amounts of liquid paraffin may deprive themselves of the fat-soluble vitamins which become dissolved in it, and may not be absorbed.

Gastric irritants, especially the antirheumatic preparations, are well known to enhance intestinal blood loss and increase the risk of iron deficiency anaemia. Other preparations such as digoxin, potassium supplements and emepronium bromide (Cetiprin) may, in some circumstances, cause gut ulceration and bleeding.

DISORDERS OF THE PANCREAS AND LIVER

Exocrine pancreatic function declines with age but not to a level where symptoms occur (Bartos and Groh, 1969; Webster et al., 1977).

When severe pancreatic pathology occurs, such as carcinoma or chronic pancreatitis, then steatorrhoea will result. The faecal fat levels may rise to levels in excess of 10 g daily. Small bowel function is however unlikely to be altered. The combination of severe steatorrhoea with a normal xylose absorption, using oral and intravenous tests together, usually indicates pancreatic disease.

Nutritional consequences are common and are frequently the presenting symptoms, especially in carcinoma of the pancreas. Anorexia, weight loss and weakness affect about one-eighth of patients at the onset of their illness, and the vast majority by the end.

Endocrine disorders of the pancreas are dealt with in Chapters 12 and 13.

Hypoalbuminaemia is well recognized as being a result of impaired hepatic function, especially in chronic conditions such as cirrhosis. In patients where an alcoholic aetiology is responsible, other nutritional defects are likely to coexist, especially folate deficiency.

Osteomalacia is also a recognized consequence of chronic liver disease (Atkinson et al., 1956), but cases seem more frequent in patients with primary biliary cirrhosis than in alcoholics.

Another group of patients with disturbed liver metabolism are those on long-term anticonvulsants. These drugs produce mitochondrial enzyme induction which leads to rapid and abnormal conversion of vitamin D (Dent et al., 1970). Calcium absorption from the gut may become impaired by the drugs (Shafer and Nuttall, 1975), probably due to reduced levels of hydroxycholecalciferol in the blood.

People with metabolic and nutritional disorders leading to hyperlipidaemia may suffer from biliary complications due to the development of cholesterol gallstones. Pancreatitis may also be precipitated by repeated attacks of cholelithiasis. These same problems can affect patients with persistent or frequently recurrent attacks of hyperbilirubinaemia. Those with haemolytic anaemias or disordered haemoglobin catabolism will develop pigment gallstones.

CHRONIC INFLAMMATORY BOWEL DISEASE

Crohn's disease and ulcerative colitis are the commonest examples of chronic inflammatory bowel disease, although tuberculous infection of the gut still occurs, but very rarely. In the elderly, ulcerative colitis is less common than in the young: McKeown (1965) found only one case in 1500 post-mortems carried out in geriatric patients. Crohn's disease would seem to be much more common in old age. As in younger patients it may predominantly affect the small bowel, and especially the terminal ileum in which case, B_{12} deficiency becomes an important feature. Large bowel involvement with Crohn's disease becomes increasingly common in the elderly (Hyams, 1974). The differentiation of ulcerative colitis and Crohn's disease therefore becomes more difficult in old age. As they may frequently occur at the same sites it is not surprising that they may both show the same nutritional consequences. Weight loss, iron deficiency anaemias, hypoproteinaemia and hypokalaemia are therefore frequent findings in Crohn's colitis (Filpsson et al., 1978) as well as in ulcerative colitis. In acute exacerbations of either, dehydration and severe electrolyte disturbances are likely to arise.

The large bowel appears to take an inconspicuous role in absorption. However, its main absorptive function is important and concerns water and electrolyte balance, hence the frequency of dehydration and hypokalaemia as complications of large bowel pathology.

CARCINOMA OF THE LARGE BOWEL

Approximately 15000 people die annually in the UK because of carcinoma of the large bowel. Over 50 per cent of these patients are elderly and the incidence increases with age. Fifty per cent of these lesions are in the rectum and 20 per cent in the sigmoid colon: obvious rectal bleeding is common, and hopefully noticed before anaemia or bowel symptoms become marked. In the 30 per cent of lesions which arise more proximally, the bleeding is more likely to be occult and anaemia becomes the common presenting symptom. It is suggested that lack of dietary fibre may play a role in the aetiology of colonic carcinoma (Cummings, 1973).

Large bowel polyps may be precancerous: in addition they make themselves obvious because of mechanical complications (e.g. intussusception) or because of excessive potassium loss leading to hypokalaemia (Schrock and Polk, 1974).

FIBRE: THE GUT AND METABOLISM

Fibre is difficult to define, but the functional description of Trowell (1972) — 'that part of the plant material taken in our diet which is resistant to digestion by the secretions of the human gastrointestinal tract' — is by far the most convenient.

After many years of being considered inert, dietary fibre is now at risk of obtaining a reputation for omnipotence. Fibre is in fact very active and its properties depend on its ability to bind other substances. It is because it can absorb and hold additional water that it is a valuable bulking agent. Stool weight is markedly increased; prolonged gut transit times shortened and rapid times decreased. Fibre is therefore potentially an ideal preparation for disordered large bowel function, especially diverticular disease and the irritable colon syndrome.

However, calcium, iron and magnesium ions may also become attached to the fibre in the bowel lumen (James et al., 1978). There is therefore considerable concern about the possibility of deficiencies of these elements being precipitated by the over-enthusiastic use of fibre supplements. The elderly may be a particularly high risk group and serum changes on high fibre diets have been recorded (Persson et al., 1976).

Fibre also has an effect on bile-salt metabolism, the excretion of salts being increased because of the interruption in their enterohepatic recirculation. Cholesterol and triglyceride levels become reduced and this has led to speculation concerning links between atherosclerosis and diet. The modern western diet is high in both refined carbohydrate and fat, but low in fibre, but it is not clear which part of this imbalance is responsible for our current diseases of affluence.

It is usually recommended that 'normal' diets should be supplemented by 20 to 30 g of bran daily (carrots, apples and oranges are good sources of fibre). However, special problems may arise in the elderly. First, this may be more than frail, ill, elderly patients are able to ingest. Secondly, although the fibre cannot be digested it can be broken down by gut flora. The colon in the elderly, especially if transit time is slow, may be colonized with large numbers of bacteria. The breakdown products of the fibre, especially free fatty acids, may cause troublesome diarrhoea. Excessive flatus production may also prove to be a problem (Davies, 1971). An additional amount of bran of 10 g daily seems to be a reasonable compromise in the elderly; the benefits of soft bulky stools and optimum transit time then occur without the disadvantage of diarrhoea (Clark and Scott, 1976).

Ten grams of fibre can be given conveniently as two slices of wholemeal bread, plus two bran biscuits plus two dessertspoonfuls of bran. If divided and spread through the day's meals this is usually managed by most patients.

REFERENCES

Andrews G. R., Haneman B., Arnold B. J. et al. (1967) *Aust. Ann. Med.* **16**, 230.
Atkinson M., Nordin B. E. C. and Sherlock S. (1956) *Q. J. Med.* **25**, 299.
Badenoch J. (1960) *Br. Med. J.* **2**, 879.
Barbezat G. O. and Grossman M. J. (1971) *Lancet* **1**, 1025.
Barry R. E., Salmon P. R., Read A. E. et al. (1971) *Gut* **12**, 873.
Bartos V. and Groh J. (1969) *Gerontol. Clin. (Basel)* **11**, 56.
Berchtold P., Dahlquist A., Gustafson A. et al. (1971) *Scand J. Gastroenterol.* **6**, 751.
Bianchi A., Chipman D. W., Dreskin A. et al. (1970) *N. Engl. J. Med.* **282**, 859.
Chalmers J. (1968) *J. R. Coll. Surg. Edinb.* **13**, 255.
Clark A. N. G. (1972) *Age Ageing* **1**, 14.

Clark A. N. G. and Scott J. F. (1976) *Age Ageing* **5**, 149.
Coghill N. F. (1969) In: Williams R. (ed.), *Chronic Idiopathic Gastritis: Causes and Effect. 5th Symposium on Advanced Medicine.* London, Pitman Medical, pp. 10–23.
Cohen T. and Gitman L. (1960) *Am. J. Gastroenterol.* **33**, 422.
Cummings J. H. (1973) *Gut* **14**, 69.
Davies P. J. (1971) *Gut* **12**, 713.
Dent C. E., Richens A., Rowe D. J. F. et al. (1970) *Br. Med. J.* **4**, 69.
Dick A. P., Graff R., Greig D. McG. et al. (1967) *Gut* **8**, 206.
Droller H. (1972) *Age Ageing* **1**, 162.
Dymock I. W., MacKay N., Miller V. et al. (1967) *Br. J. Cancer* **21**, 505.
Elkeles A. (1964) *Am. J. Roetgenol.* **91**, 744.
Falaiye J. M. (1971) *Br. Med. J.* **4**, 454.
Filpsson S., Hulten L., Lindstedt G. et al. (1978) *Scand. J. Gastroenterol.* **13**, 471.
Foroozan P. and Trier J. S. (1967) *N. Engl. J. Med.* **277**, 553.
Gerson C. D. G. W., Hepner N., Brown A. et al. (1972) *Gastroenterol.* **63**, 246.
Gough K. R., Read A. E. and Naish J. M. (1962) *Gut* **3**, 232.
Hermos J. A., Adams W. H., Liu Y. K. et al. (1972) *Ann. Intern. Med.* **76**, 957.
Hyams D. E. (1974) *Br. Med. J.* **2**, 150.
Hyde R. D. and Loehry C. A. E. H. (1968) *Gut* **9**, 717.
Ikkala E., Salmi H. J. and Siurala M. (1970) *Acta Haematol.* **43**, 228.
James W. P. T., Branch W. I. and Southgate D. A. T. (1978) *Lancet* **1**, 638.
Jones A. W., Kirk R. S. and Bloor K. (1970) *Gut* **11**, 679.
Joske R. A. and Blackwell J. B. (1959) *Lancet* **2**, 379.
Jounela A. J., Pirittiaho H. and Palva I. P. (1974) *Acta Med. Scand.* **196**, 267.
Katz J. H., Dimase J. and Donaldson R. M. (1963) *J. Lab. Clin. Med.* **61**, 266.
Kendall M. J. (1970) *Gut* **11**, 498.
Kendall M. J. and Nutter S. (1970) *Gut* **11**, 1020.
McBrien D. J. and Lockhart-Mummery H. E. (1962) *Br. Med. J.* **2**, 1653.
McGuigan J. E. and Trudeau W. L. (1968) *N. Engl. J. Med.* **278**, 1308.
McKeown F. (1965) *Pathology of the Aged.* London, Butterworths.
Marks J. and Shuster S. (1968) *Br. Med. J.* **4**, 455.
Milledge J. S. (1972) *Br. Med. J.* **3**, 557.
Morson B. C. (1955) *Br. J. Cancer* **9**, 365.
Mosbech J. and Videbaek A. (1950) *Br. Med. J.* **2**, 390.
Murray J. S., Paton R. P. and Pope C. E. (1961) *N. Engl. J. Med.* **264**, 436.
Naqvi M. S., Burrows L. and Kark A. E. (1969) *Ann. Surg.* **170**, 221.
Pelz K. S., Gottfried S. P. and Soos E. (1968) *Geriatrics* **23**, 149.
Persson I., Raby K., Fønss-Bech P. et al. (1976) *J. Am. Geriatr. Soc.* **7**, 334.
Pettersson T., Wegelius O. and Skrifuars B. (1970) *Acta Med. Scand.* **188**, 139.
Price H. L., Gazzard B. G. and Dawson A. M. (1977) *Br. Med. J.* **1**, 1582.
Rath C. E., McCurdy P. R. and Duffy B. J. (1957) *N. Engl. J. Med.* **256**, 111.
Reynolds E. H., Milner G., Matthews D. M. et al. (1966) *Q. J. Med.* **35**, 521.
Rosenberg I. H., Streiff R. R., Godwin H. A. et al. (1969) *N. Engl. J. Med.* **280**, 985.
Saraya A. K., Tandon B. N., Ramachandran K. et al. (1971) *Am. J. Clin. Nutr.* **24**, 622.
Schrock L. G. and Polk H. C. jun. (1974) *Am. Surg.* **40**, 54.
Scott G. B., Williams M. J. and Clark C. G. (1964) *Gut* **5**, 553.
Shafer R. B. and Nuttall F. Q. (1975) *J. Clin. Endocrinol. Metab.* **41**, 1125.
Siurala M. and Seppala K. (1960) *Acta Med. Scand.* **166**, 455.
Stalsberg H. and Taksdal S. (1971) *Lancet* **2**, 1175.
Stowers J. M. and Bewsher P. D. (1969) *Postgrad. Med. J.* Suppl. **45**, 13.
Summerskill W. H. J. (1959) *Lancet* **1**, 120.
Trowell H. C. (1972) *Atherosclerosis* **16**, 138.

Varito T. (1962) *Scand. J. Clin. Lab. Invest.* **14**, 36.

Waldmann T. A. (1970) In: Card W. I. and Creamer B. (ed.), *Modern Trends in Gastroenterology*. London, Butterworths, pp. 125–142.

Webster S. G. P. (1973) MD Thesis. University of London.

Webster S. G. P. and Leeming J. T. (1975a) *Age Ageing* **4**, 168.

Webster S. G. P. and Leeming J. T. (1975b) *Gut* **16**, 109.

Webster S. G. P., Wilkinson E. M. and Gowland E. (1977) *Age and Ageing* **6**, 113.

Zollinger R. M. and Ellison E. H. (1955) *Ann. Surg.* **142**, 709.

10. NUTRITION AND ANAEMIA
D. E. Hyams

The World Health Organization defines anaemia as a condition in which the haemoglobin concentration, or the haematocrit, or the number of red blood cells is below the level which is normal for a given individual (WHO, 1972). The 'normal' haemoglobin concentration is difficult to define; it will vary with age, sex, weight, psychological status and altitude. In any community the distribution of haemoglobin concentration in anaemic persons overlaps that for persons with normal haemoglobin concentrations (Pryce, 1960). Nevertheless, WHO has made recommendations regarding the haemoglobin levels below which anaemia may be considered to be present (WHO, 1968; 1972). These values (which apply at sea-level) may be taken as 13 g/dl for adult males and 12 g/dl for adult non-pregnant females. Normal old people are not by definition anaemic and the same criteria should be adopted for them (Hyams, 1973).

Nutritional anaemia is anaemia due to a deficiency of one or more essential nutrients, regardless of the cause of that deficiency (WHO, 1968). An inadequate supply of one or more of these haemopoietic nutrients leads to inability of erythropoietic tissue to maintain a normal haemoglobin concentration (Layrisse et al., 1976), but nutritional factors other than specific deficiencies may also play a part in the development of anaemia.

INCIDENCE OF NUTRITIONAL ANAEMIAS
Although it is accepted that nutritional anaemias affect large population groups in developing countries (WHO, 1968), many developed countries also have a high prevalence of nutritional anaemias in certain groups of the population (e.g. children and women of childbearing age). Iron deficiency is by far the commonest nutritional disorder, as well as the commonest cause of anaemia. Folate deficiency ranks second as a cause of nutritional anaemia (WHO, 1975). Dietary deficiency of vitamin B_{12} is very much less common (Baker, 1967) and anaemia is a late development in patients with protein deficiency (Viteri et al., 1968).

It is difficult to obtain reliable figures for the incidence of anaemia due solely to nutritional factors in the elderly. Old people are undoubtedly vulnerable to dietary inadequacies (Exton-Smith, 1977), and many elderly persons have blood and tissue levels of nutrients which are below the normal levels for younger age groups; yet low dietary intakes and abnormal biochemical findings are rarely associated with clinical evidence of malnutrition (Exton-Smith, 1977; Attwood et al., 1978). Frank anaemia due to nutritional deficiency alone seems relatively uncommon in old age, though nutritional factors often play some part in the pathogenesis of anaemia in elderly patients. For example, iron-deficiency anaemia in old people is more often associated with chronic gastrointestinal blood loss than with inadequate iron intake alone (Bedford and Wollner, 1958); however, both factors are frequently implicated. Folic acid deficiency is common in the elderly, but anaemia due solely to folic acid deficiency is not common (Batata et al., 1967; Evans et al., 1968; Ellwood et al., 1971; DHSS, 1972; MacLennan et al., 1973). Dietary deficiency of vitamin B_{12} is seen in vegans (Stewart et al., 1970), but elderly vegans are relatively rare.

PREDISPOSING FACTORS
Exton-Smith (1977) has described the primary and secondary causes of malnutrition in the elderly. Ageing may lead to defects in smell and taste which may in turn be associated with loss of appetite. This, together with increased difficulty in obtaining and preparing food, acts to reduce dietary intake at a time of life when certain requirements may actually be increased (because of low body stores, for example, resulting from chronic blood loss or long-standing dietary inadequacies).

The Gastrointestinal System
Inefficient mastication due to the edentulous state or inadequate dentures may lead to a conditioned deficiency (*see* p. 102) since it leads to the consumption of a soft diet which is likely to be unbalanced and unappetizing. Nevertheless, there is no good evidence of an association between dental state and any clinically important nutritional deficiency (Neill, 1972; Hubbard-Ryland, 1973).

The incidence of gastric mucosal abnormalities is said to increase with advancing age (Joske et al., 1955), although this has been contested by Bird et al. (1977). Nevertheless, the incidence of parietal cell antibodies in the serum increases after the age of 60 (Doniach and Roitt, 1964; Wangel et al., 1968). The incidence of achlorhydria also increases with advancing age (Vanzant et al., 1932; Polland, 1933; Edwards and Coghill, 1966; Wangel et al., 1968) and this may reduce the efficiency of iron absorption (McCurdy and Dern, 1968).

There may also be a physiological decrease in the absorption of nutrients in old age. This has been reported for iron (Bonnet et al., 1960; Freiman et al., 1963; Vancini et al., 1967; Jacobs and Owen, 1969) and calcium (Nordin et al., 1976). Webster and Leeming (1975) showed that proximal jejunal villi tended to be broader and shorter in old than in young subjects; however, the old subjects all had normal red-cell folate levels, suggesting that they were not suffering from malnutrition which might have influenced the appearance of the small bowel mucosa (Barry et al., 1971). Some early reports of diminished vitamin B_{12} absorption in old age have not been confirmed (Hyams, 1964; 1973). However iron status may affect vitamin B_{12} absorption (Cox et al., 1959).

Folate absorption is not affected by ageing, but dietary deficiency of folate appears to induce a reversible impairment of folic acid absorption (Elsborg, 1976).

The liver content of vitamin B_{12} is not decreased in old age (Swendseid et al., 1954; Halsted et al., 1959). Thus normal old people do not have depleted vitamin B_{12}.

'CONDITIONED' DEFICIENCY OF NUTRIENTS

Drugs may affect the supply or utilization of haemopoietic nutrients in several ways: for example, loss of iron (gastrointestinal bleeding); impaired absorption [pH change, e.g. due to cimetidine (Esposito, 1977)] ; impaired utilization of iron (drug-induced sideroblastic anaemia); or folic acid deficiency (anticonvulsants, folic acid antagonists, sulphasalazine) (Franklin and Rosenberg, 1973; Schneider and Beeley, 1977).

Alcohol can produce iron deficiency by replacing normal food intake or by inducing lesions of the gastrointestinal tract which bleed. Alcohol can produce folic acid deficiency (Wu et al., 1975) by replacing normal food intake, or by impairing hepatic function. Combined iron and folic acid deficiencies may occur (Green and Trowbridge, 1977). Alcohol may also have a direct depressant effect on the bone marrow (Editorial, *Lancet*, 1977b; Myrhed et al., 1977) and has been shown to be toxic to red-cell precursors in the absence of folic acid deficiency (Lindenbaum and Lieber, 1969). Macrocytosis has been attributed to alcohol in the absence of folate or vitamin B_{12} deficiency (Wu et al., 1974; Editorial, *Br. Med. J.*, 1978).

Food (e.g. wholemeal bread) may inhibit absorption of non-haem iron (Dobbs and Baird, 1977). Other causes of gastrointestinal bleeding and uterine bleeding are important causes of iron deficiency.

INFLUENCE OF NUTRITION ON OTHER ANAEMIAS

Multiple pathology is the rule in elderly patients; poor nutritional status may aggravate the degree or effect of anaemia due to other causes; these include drug-related anaemias (Basu, 1977).

Nutritional deficiencies are often multiple, and anaemia may include more than one nutritional deficiency in its pathogenesis. In particular, combined deficiency of iron and folic acid is not rare, and iron-deficiency anaemia may coexist with pernicious anaemia. These mixed-aetiology anaemias may present a dimorphic peripheral blood picture, and iron deficiency may prevent the appearance of megaloblastic changes in the bone marrow; when the iron deficiency is corrected the megaloblastic change is unmasked, but if not sought at that time it may be missed.

IRON-DEFICIENCY ANAEMIA
Iron Requirements

Iron requirements in healthy adults have been considered to be 0·6 mg daily (WHO, 1968), since this is the estimated mean daily loss in the absence of disease. Recommended iron intake has been given as 10 mg per day in old age, for both sexes, to allow a wide margin of safety (DHSS, 1969; WHO, 1970). Actual intake may often be less than this, as it tends to fall with age (Hallberg and Högdahl, 1971). In a national nutritional survey of 879 old people aged 65 and over living at home (DHSS, 1972), the daily mean iron intake was 10·2 mg; but only the men had values above 10 mg. Average values for women were 9·4 mg per day in 65–74 years age group and only 8·5 mg per day in the age group 75 years and over. In a study of the diet of elderly women living alone (Exton-Smith and Stanton, 1965), 60 women had a daily mean iron intake of 9·9 mg. In 16 of the women, when this study was followed up seven years later, the daily mean iron intake had fallen to 8·9 (Stanton and Exton-Smith, 1970). However, when iron intake is related to energy intake, the differences disappear. MacLennan et al. (1973) found similar values for daily intakes of iron in their survey of 475 elderly people living at home; they noted, however, that subjects with iron deficiency and anaemia did not on average take less iron than those with neither condition.

Iron absorption increases when body stores fall or when erythropoiesis is stimulated. It may be increased by simultaneous administration of vitamin C (McCurdy and Dern, 1968). Much work has been carried out on the absorption of iron from foodstuffs (Layrisse, 1975; WHO, 1975). Old peoples' iron intake derives mainly from meat, flour products and eggs. Whereas iron absorption may be up to 25 per cent from meat, it is below 10 per cent from vegetable foods, in some cases less than one per cent (WHO, 1975). The phytate in wheat bran inhibits iron absorption (Björn-Rasmussen, 1974), an important matter when regular bran consumption is advocated (Cleave et al., 1969). Other foods which inhibit iron absorption are eggs, milk, and tea (Callender, 1971; Disler et al., 1975), all of which are important items in the diet of elderly people.

Iron Transport

Plasma iron and total iron-binding capacity (TIBC) fall with ageing; plasma iron starts to fall after 30 years of age and TIBC after 50 years (Powell and Thomas, 1969). Plasma iron may rise again in women after 60 (Thomas, 1971), so that the sex difference in plasma iron levels seen at earlier years disappears. There is no sex difference in TIBC levels.

Iron is transported in plasma in combination with a protein (transferrin) which is decreased in old age (Weeks and Krasilnikoff, 1972). Transferrin is normally one-third saturated with iron, but the range may be wide in the elderly (MacLennan et al., 1973). This test reflects the adequacy of iron supplies to the bone marrow, but is labile and not always a reliable index of iron deficiency. A more stringent interpretation (one-sixth saturation) correlates better with iron deficiency (Mitchell and Pegrum, 1971). Plasma iron and transferrin saturation do not correlate well with haemoglobin levels (Powell et al., 1968), but show significant correlation with mean corpuscular haemoglobin concentration (MCHC) (Powell et al., 1968; Evans, 1971).

Average normal adult values are given as:

	Plasma Iron	TIBC
Men	23 μmol/l (125 μg/dl) ⎱	53–71 μmol/l
Women	20 μmol/l (110 μg/dl) ⎰	300–400 μg/dl

Normal levels in old age are uncertain: levels of plasma iron as low as 9 μmol/l (50 μg/dl) may occur in the presence of normal iron stores, and values of 11–14 μmol/l (60–80 μg/dl) without anaemia are not uncommon. Thus plasma iron levels must be considered together with TIBC and percentage transferrin saturation in the assessment of iron status. In true iron deficiency the TIBC rises and saturation falls. Where available, serum ferritin estimations may be very helpful (see below).

Iron Utilization
Refractory iron-deficiency anaemia may be due to impaired utilization of iron by the bone marrow, rather than a true shortage of body iron. Examples are the 'anaemias of chronic disorders' (Cartwright, 1966; Turnbull, 1971), sideroblastic anaemias (see p. 109) and transferrin deficiency, e.g. due to impaired protein synthesis (Heilmeyer, 1966).

Iron Stores
There are two storage forms of iron: haemosiderin and ferritin. Both forms increase in the bone marrow with increasing age, and at all ages men have more than women (Burkhardt, 1975). Haemosiderin is stainable in the reticulo-endothelial cells. Ferritin is soluble and is estimated chemically or visualized on electron microscopy. Until recently, ferritin was considered an intracellular protein which entered the plasma only after cellular necrosis; however, it is now known that ferritin reflects iron stores (Jacobs, 1975), correlating approximately with the amount of stainable iron in the bone marrow (Hussein et al., 1975). Normal values of serum ferritin in adults are 12–300 μg/l of serum. There is a progressive increase with age after 20 years in men, and after the menopause in women (Cook, 1975), but there is no sex difference in old age.

Iron Loss

Physiological losses of iron in the elderly total about 14 mg/day/kg body weight (WHO, 1970), mainly as faecal iron. Pathological iron loss comes mainly from the gastrointestinal tract. Occult gastrointestinal bleeding is common in the elderly (Bedford and Wollner, 1958), and even when tests for faecal occult blood are negative, there may be appreciable blood loss from gastrointestinal lesions such as hiatus hernia or after partial gastrectomy (Holt et al., 1968; 1970). Haemorrhoids are common, and large bowel carcinoma should never be forgotten. Regular ingestion of salicylates may cause chronic blood loss (Scott et al., 1961), and this is not uncommon as a cause of iron deficiency and anaemia in the elderly (MacLennan et al., 1973). Vitamin C deficiency is said to predispose to gastrointestinal bleeding after salicylate ingestion. Other drugs may also lead to gastrointestinal bleeding. Bleeding from other sources is a rarer cause of iron-deficiency anaemia (e.g. haematuria, haemoptyses, epistaxes, uterine bleeding).

Effects of Iron Deficiency

1. *On Tissues*

These are reviewed by Dallman (1974). Atrophic glossitis, angular stomatitis and atrophic changes in the buccal mucosa have been described, but some of these may be due to concomitant vitamin B deficiency. Koilonychia may occur, with or without other features of the Plummer—Vinson syndrome: an oesophageal web is rare but is a premalignant condition. Gastric mucosal abnormalities are common but do not correlate with the degree of anaemia. Gastric atrophy develops gradually and there is loss of ability to secrete hydrochloric acid, pepsin and intrinsic factor, in that order (Witts, 1966). Achlorhydria may commonly occur even with normal gastric mucosa (Bird et al., 1977). Gastric parietal-cell antibodies are not uncommon in patients with iron deficiency, and the prevalence of these antibodies increases with age (Wangel et al., 1968). These autoantibodies may further damage the gastric mucosa (Anderson et al., 1967; Walder, 1968). Peripheral neuropathy may develop.

2. *On the Body*

Resistance to infection may be diminished because of impaired activity of enzymes in granulocytes and/or reduction in immune response (WHO, 1975; Strauss, 1978). Drug metabolism may be altered in iron deficiency: antipyrine metabolism was more rapid in six iron-deficient subjects aged over 65 years who were free of renal, hepatic or gastrointestinal disease and who were not taking drugs known to influence hepatic microsomal enzymes (Langman and Smithard, 1977).

Clinical Features

Standard texts may be consulted for a full account of the clinical features of iron-deficiency anaemia, but some aspects of particular relevance in the elderly will be considered here. Patients may be symptomless, or may attribute symptoms to old age and so fail to bring them to the attention of their family or to seek medical advice. This is especially likely if the onset of the anaemia is insidious. By the time the anaemia is diagnosed the patient may be very ill indeed. Where there are symptoms, cardiovascular and cerebral manifestations predominate: breathlessness, ankle swelling, frank congestive cardiac failure or left ventricular failure, dizziness, non-specific mental deterioration with confusion, and perhaps apathy or agitation. There may be delusions or hallucinations. Pallor of mucosae or nail beds is a more useful sign than pallor of skin.

Diagnosis

The characteristic blood picture of iron-deficiency anaemia is that of a hypochromic anaemia which soon becomes microcytic, with anisocytosis and poikilocytosis; but the peripheral blood picture alone is not a reliable index of iron deficiency. Standard texts may be consulted for a full account of the blood, bone marrow, biochemical changes and radio-isotope test findings in iron-deficiency anaemia. The presence of anaemia must lead to an evaluation of its cause and a search for any underlying condition. A full blood count, MCHC, plasma iron and TIBC usually allow a diagnosis of iron-deficiency anaemia, and its cause must then be found.

A full medical history, including details of drug ingestion or gastric operation, must be supplemented by information on the diet and food habits of the patients — though reliable information on this point may be difficult to obtain (*see* Chapter 6). Non-nutritional factors must always be sought for, and other possible causes of iron-deficiency vigorously excluded. A full examination will include proctoscopy. Faecal occult blood tests are mandatory and barium studies and/or sigmoidoscopy may be needed. More specialized investigations may also be appropriate.

Always search for other coexisting causes of anaemia. Dagg et al. (1964) estimated that a patient with iron-deficiency anaemia and achlorhydria has a 32 per cent chance of developing pernicious anaemia. Other nutritional deficiencies (e.g. of folic acid or vitamin C) may coexist.

Treatment

The deficiency of iron must be made good, including the replenishment of iron stores. This simple requirement is beset with many potential problems, especially in the elderly.

Many patients will stop treatment when they feel better, and this makes it difficult to continue their iron replacement for a period long enough to replenish body stores, i.e. 3 to 6 months longer than the patient thinks necessary, or longer if chronic blood loss cannot be stopped, or the diet improved. This may be a particular problem in the elderly, who may in any case find it difficult to remember to take iron tablets regularly.

1. *Oral Iron Therapy*

Oral iron therapy is used in every case unless contraindicated. One 200 mg tablet of ferrous sulphate (the simplest and cheapest form of therapy) provides 60 mg elemental iron and in anaemia about one-third of this can be absorbed. However, not more than 20—60 mg iron can be absorbed in a day (Coleman et al., 1955), so that it is unnecessary to insist on thrice daily dosage in all cases. This consideration is of relevance to treatment of the elderly, and it is doubtful whether there is any need to prefer slow-release iron preparations on the grounds that they may be taken less often; they offer no other advantage (Callender, 1969; Ellwood and Williams, 1970).

Side-effects of oral iron therapy are related to the dose of elemental iron ingested — another reason for keeping dosage as low as possible. The tablet should be given after a meal and, if side-effects do appear, ferrous gluconate, fumarate or succinate may be tried instead of ferrous sulphate. If preferred, a liquid iron preparation may be used, but since these present the iron in ferric form a daily intake of 1000 mg elemental iron is required.

In general, iron should be given alone; the only exception is the possible concomitant administration of vitamin C or succinic acid to increase its absorption. Vitamin C increases the incidence of side-effects of iron (Witts, 1969), and succinic acid is to be preferred (Hallberg and Sölvell, 1966) — if indeed, any such adjuvant is really needed at all.

Parenteral iron therapy will be required where there is malabsorption, or where oral iron therapy is considered undesirable or impracticable. Witts (1969) gives a formula for the approximate amount of iron required to be injected to correct anaemia and replenish body iron stores:

$$\text{mg iron to be injected} = (15 - \text{patient's haemoglobin in g per 100 ml}) \times \text{body weight in kg} \times 3.$$

2. *Intramuscular Iron*

Iron-dextran injection (Imferon) or iron-sorbitol injection (Jectofer) may be used by intramuscular injection. Each contains 50 mg iron per ml. Imferon may be used intramuscularly in the elderly but must be injected deeply to avoid skin staining; it may produce local tenderness and lymphadenopathy. A test dose of 1 ml is followed by 2 ml doses from 1 to 3 days apart, increasing up to 5 ml if tolerated. Imferon should be avoided in uraemic patients. Jectofer does not stain skin and rarely produces local symptoms or signs. Doses should not exceed 2 ml daily and must never be given intravenously. Oral iron should not be given during Jectofer therapy, since toxic effects have been produced in this way. Side-effects of intramuscular iron include local reactions as described and general reactions resembling (but less frequent than) those seen with intravenous iron (*see* p. 108).

A new preparation of iron for intramuscular use currently under investigation and showing considerable promise is iron-poly (sorbitol-gluconic acid) complex. (Ferastral). This is a development arising from

Jectofer (Fielding, 1977). Evers (1977) reported that the response to intramuscular Ferastral is as good as the response to total dose intravenous infusion of Imferon, in comparable patients. A limited experience has so far been reported in the elderly, and this has been satisfactory (Olsson, 1977; Sundin, 1977).

3. Intravenous Iron

Saccharated iron oxide (Ferrivenin) or iron-dextrin (formerly Astrafer IV) are for intravenous use only. The former is more irritant and more likely to produce local and general reactions than the latter.

Total-dose iron infusions are time-saving and reasonably safe if applied with care. Wright (1967) and Andrews et al. (1967) advocated their use in the elderly. Imferon is given in saline (possibly with 40 mg frusemide added to ensure a diuresis) at a slow rate, so that 1 litre fluid is infused over 4—6 hours. The initial rate of flow is kept at 10 drops per minute for 10—30 minutes, as a test dose, then increased to 45—60 drops per minute. The patient is observed for at least one hour after the end of the infusion: the procedure is thus suitable for day hospital use (Andrews et al., 1967).

Local irritation, venous spasm or phlebitis may occur. General reactions give rise to symptoms such as nausea, vomiting, fever, tachycardia, and head and abdominal pain. Hypersensitivity, anaphylactoid reactions and anuria have been reported. Reactions to Ferrivenin were reported in 5—35 per cent of patients by Coleman et al. (1955). Total dose infusion has given severe reactions in 0—6 per cent of patients, with a higher incidence of milder reactions. Intravenous iron therapy gives fewer reactions in severe iron-deficiency, presumably due to increased plasma iron-binding capacity.

4. Blood Transfusion

Blood transfusion is rarely required in iron-deficiency anaemia unless there is acute severe blood loss. In chronic anaemias the blood volume is maintained or increased, and sudden further increase by blood transfusion (even packed cells) may be very hazardous.

Prevention

Education of the public (not only the elderly) will help to prevent the development of iron deficiency. Such education needs to incorporate not only information on the iron content of various foods but also modern knowledge on the absorption of food iron and inhibitory factors in the diet. This is especially important for the elderly, although it must be recognized that old people may resist changes in their dietary habits.

Education may be given via public media, schools (for children and adults), old peoples' clubs, voluntary organizations, day hospitals, and by health visitors and doctors on an individual basis. It should also be included in pre-retirement courses.

Full use should be made of dietitians and nutritionists in these educative endeavours. The social worker and health visitor can also help to ensure that the elderly are aware of the importance of these aspects of diet and health, and of the availability of further education in these matters.

On a larger scale, the question of fortification of foods with iron must be considered. Several countries (e.g. Sweden, the UK, and the USA) have programmes in operation for the fortification of wheat flour with iron (WHO, 1975; Crosby, 1978).

No fortification programme has been specifically directed at the elderly as a vulnerable group, and it is perhaps doubtful whether this would be feasible. However, the Panel on Nutrition of the Elderly (DHSS, 1972) recommended a study of the possibility of using milk fortified with several nutrients for vulnerable groups (e.g. as an extension of the meals-on-wheels or luncheon clubs service or as a separate project).

Prevention of pathological iron loss is also of paramount importance.

LATENT IRON DEFICIENCY

Iron deficiency without anaemia is common in the elderly (Batata et al., 1967; McFarlane et al., 1967; Jacobs et al., 1969; Lloyd, 1971; Mitchell and Pegrum, 1971; Thomas and Powell, 1971). MacLennan et al. (1973) found this condition to be commoner than iron deficiency with anaemia in their community study. If the deficiency persists, anaemia is likely to follow; this situation is analogous to latent pernicious anaemia.

SIDEROBLASTIC ANAEMIA

This refractory anaemia is associated with impaired utilization of iron and hyperplastic bone marrow containing ring sideroblasts. The proximate cause is a defect in porphyrin synthesis, which may be hereditary or acquired. When seen in old age the anaemia is acquired, but may be primary or secondary. Folic acid deficiency often coexists, with a megaloblastic marrow, but folate repletion does not always correct the megaloblastosis. Secondary sideroblastic anaemia may occur in association with diseases impairing nutrition (e.g. malabsorption, alcoholism, partial gastrectomy, neoplasm), or as part of the picture of other blood diseases, or as a manifestation of drug toxicity (antituberculous drugs, paracetamol, cytotoxic agents).

Folic acid and/or vitamin B_{12} may help; remission may be complete in the secondary forms. Pyridoxine has sometimes been successful even in the absence of evidence of vitamin B_6 deficiency. A therapeutic trial is worthwhile, although Israels (1975) considers that the elderly do not respond. Mason and Emerson (1973) were successful in treating sideroblastic anaemia in a 72-year-old woman with pyridoxal-5'-phosphate; but very few of the elderly patients described by Trump et al. (1975) responded to this treatment, even though several had decreased amino-laevulinic acid synthetase activity. Vitamin C may be of some help, especially if given with chelating agents (Wapnick et al., 1969). Phlebotomy has been used to reduce body iron; blood transfusions greatly increase the risk of iron overload and liver damage.

MEGALOBLASTIC ANAEMIAS
Megaloblastic anaemias are macrocytic anaemias with oversized and abnormal red-cell precursors (megaloblasts) in the bone marrow. Leucopenia and a tendency to hypersegmentation of neutrophil nuclei are common features. The incidence of these anaemias increases with age, and they may produce severe illness in the elderly because of late diagnosis. However, most megaloblastic anaemias are treatable and it is important to make the diagnosis before complications ensue which may be far less amenable to medical intervention.

Folic Acid — Vitamin B_{12} Interrelationships
Megaloblastic anaemias are deficiency diseases due usually to lack of vitamin B_{12} or folic acid; deficiency of either of these nutrients leads to defective nucleic acid synthesis, which leads in turn to megaloblastosis in the marrow. Peripheral blood changes follow.

The immediate cause of the defect in nucleic acid synthesis is folate deficiency. In body fluids, folate is 5-methyltetrahydrofolate (5-methyl THF) which acts as a methyl-donor in the conversion of homocysteine to methionine by the enzyme tetrahydrofolic methyltransferase (EC2.1.1.13). Vitamin B_{12} is a coenzyme in this reaction.

In vitamin B_{12} deficiency the transmethylation reaction is interfered with and 5-methyl THF is thought to accumulate ('methyltrap' hypothesis; Herbert and Zalusky, 1962; Noronha and Silverman, 1962). Despite some evidence to the contrary (Chanarin, 1973, 1974; Perry et al., 1976), this hypothesis is still widely considered to be the most satisfactory explanation for the relationship between folic acid, vitamin B_{12} and methionine (Shin et al., 1975; Das and Herbert, 1976; Zittoun et al., 1978).

FOLIC ACID DEFICIENCY
Folic Acid Requirements and Recommended Allowance
The minimal daily requirement of folic acid (as pteroylmonoglutamic acid, PGA) is 50—100 μg, but when there is increased erythropoiesis the need may be as much as 1 mg daily. The recommended daily allowance is 200 μg PGA for adults (WHO, 1970; Passmore et al., 1974). Since normal diets contain both 'free' (PGA) and 'bound' (polyglutamate) folate in approximately equal amounts, and it is now thought that polyglutamates in foodstuffs are effectively deconjugated to monoglutamates during absorption (WHO, 1975), the recommended daily dietary allowance of folic acid has also been stated as 400 μg 'total' folate (WHO, 1972; NAS/NRC, 1974; Harper, 1978); (but see comments under *folic acid absorption* below).

An average mixed diet contains 500–800 μg total folate per day. In the elderly, however, there is much evidence of inadequate dietary intake of folate (Gough et al., 1963; Forshaw et al., 1964; Read et al., 1965; Exton-Smith and Stanton, 1965; Girdwood, 1969; MacLennan et al., 1973). Forshaw et al. (1964) reported 17 patients, all aged over 60 years, who had megaloblastic anaemia due to a dietary folate deficiency. MacLennan et al. (1973) found low folate intakes to be common, but only rarely was this reflected in evidence of folate deficiency; in particular, anaemia due to this cause was extremely uncommon, and in each instance there was associated iron deficiency.

Folic Acid Absorption and Malabsorption
Folic acid absorption as PGA is not affected by ageing but it may be impaired in conditions of nutritional deficiency, returning to normal after folic acid therapy (Elsborg, 1976). Folic acid deficiency has been reported to cause cellular changes in the upper jejunal epithelium (Berg et al., 1972; Bianchi et al., 1970; Editorial, *Lancet*, 1977a).

Absorption of folates from dietary sources may not be as effective in the elderly as in the young. Baker at al. (1978) showed that elderly subjects absorbed folates very poorly from yeast, in contrast to their efficient absorption of riboflavin, vitamin B_6 and pantothenate from yeast and their efficient absorption of synthetic folylmonoglutamate. In younger control subjects yeast was a significant folate source. These authors suggested that the enzyme folate conjugase, secreted mainly by small intestinal mucosa (Rosenberg, 1976), and the means by which polyglutamates are converted to monoglutamates during absorption, may be decreased in old age. Common causes of malabsorption include gluten-sensitive enteropathy and tropical sprue, both of which are important causes of folate deficiency.

Folic Acid Utilization
Increased cell-turnover (especially of primitive cells) calls for increased amounts of folate, up to 10 times normal. Increased utilization also occurs in infections, chronic inflammatory diseases, rheumatoid arthritis, and thyrotoxicosis. Impaired utilization may occur in vitamin C deficiency, since vitamin C maintains folate coenzymes in their reduced active state (Cox, 1968; Chanarin, 1969; Booth and Todd, 1970). Megaloblastic anaemia may result (Goldberg, 1963; Hyams and Ross, 1963; Vilter, 1964; Cox, 1968).

Clinical Features
Mental changes may occur with folic acid deficiency, and may be mild and non-specific (Editorial, *Lancet*, 1969). A possible association between dementia and folate deficiency (Strachan and Henderson, 1967; Sneath et al., 1973) was not confirmed by Shaw (1971) or MacLennan et al. (1973).

Neurological features include a picture resembling subacute combined degeneration of the cord; early treatment with folic acid can reverse neurological damage (Pincus et al., 1972; Manzoor and Runcie, 1976). It is mandatory to exclude concomitant vitamin B_{12} deficiency, since administration of folic acid alone in such cases could precipitate or aggravate the neurological changes. For a more detailed discussion, see Editorial, *Br. Med. J.* and *Lancet* (1976), and Reynolds (1976a, b).

Diagnosis

When anaemia develops it has the typical features of megaloblastic anaemia, indistinguishable from that due to vitamin B_{12} deficiency. Macrocytosis may precede other evidence of folate deficiency; 18 out of 40 elderly patients with macrocytosis developed folic acid deficiency over the next six months (Raper and Choudhury, 1978).

Serum folate is usually below 2 or 3 ng/ml in folate deficiency, and often less than 1 ng/ml if anaemia is present. It is difficult to decide on the normal range of serum folate in old age; it is probably best to accept 2·5 or 3 ng/ml as normal (Thomas and Powell, 1971), rather than the formerly accepted range of 6–21 ng/ml (Wintrobe, 1967). Serum folate responds rapidly to changes in dietary intake of folate. Red cells have a life of 3–4 months and red-cell folate thus affords a better idea of the dietary habits and folate stores of the patient (Hoffbrand et al., 1966). Other tests include the FIGLU test and folate absorption and clearance tests (Chanarin, 1969), and the deoxyuridine suppression test (Wickramasinghe and Longland, 1974; Zittoun et al., 1978). A liver biopsy may be assayed for folate (Pitney and Onesti, 1961).

Despite the use of such tests there may still be doubt about the diagnosis. In this case a haematological response may be sought after very small oral doses of folic acid: in true folate deficiency a daily dose of 200–500 μg will produce an optimal response.

Treatment

Folic acid is given orally, 10–20 mg daily, reducing to 2·5–10 mg daily for maintenance. If there is malabsorption or very severe anaemia, folic acid may be injected as the sodium salt, 15 mg daily, reducing to 5–10 mg daily.

If vitamin B_{12} deficiency has not been excluded, it is dangerous to give folic acid alone. Epileptics given folic acid may lose control of fits.

Blood transfusion should be reserved for crises during the course of severe anaemia. Packed cells should be used, with precautions against fluid overload in elderly patients (small volumes at slow rates, addition of a diuretic, warming of veins, and careful clinical observation).

Prevention of Folate Deficiency

It has now become routine, in many parts of the world, to provide prophylactic folic acid supplementation for pregnant women. It is less easy to introduce folic acid supplementation of the diets of elderly people, for reasons already given. Although Read et al. (1965) suggested that 25–50 μg doses of folic acid should be given to elderly people living alone, it is quite likely that such small amounts will not be absorbed if folic acid deficiency is already present (Elsborg, 1976). Furthermore, administration of folic acid in a 'blind' or 'blanket' manner could lead to neurological or other problems in certain instances (Batata et al., 1967). It is preferable for professional deliverers of health care to have a high awareness of the likelihood of folate deficiency in the elderly and to act accordingly to prevent or to investigate and treat appropriately in each individual case.

VITAMIN B_{12} DEFICIENCY

The body loses 0·1 per cent of its total vitamin B_{12} daily. Passmore et al. (1974) give the daily B_{12} loss as 0·25 μg to 1·0 μg, but other authorities report losses of up to 7·8 μg daily.

The recommended allowance (WHO, 1970) of B_{12} is 2 μg daily (after 10 years of age); in the elderly this would appear to be on the low side. The American recommendation (NAS/NRC, 1974) is 3 μg daily after the age of 51 years (Harper, 1978). Nevertheless, dietary deficiency of B_{12} is excessively rare except in vegans, and even in them the signs and symptoms of vitamin B_{12} deficiency are uncommon (Chanarin, 1969).

Vitamin B_{12} Intake

Vitamin B_{12} is found in all foods of animal origin; milk, eggs and meat are important sources. Vegetable foods contain virtually no B_{12}. A normal diet contains up to 30 μg vitamin B_{12} daily — larger amounts in the USA, less in the UK.

Vitamin B_{12} Absorption and Malabsorption

Under physiological conditions, absorption of vitamin B_{12} takes place only after the vitamin is bound to a mucoprotein secreted by gastric parietal cells — intrinsic factor (IF). The IF–B_{12} complex is absorbed in the ileum. No more than 2–3 μg of vitamin B_{12} can be absorbed from a single meal; daily absorption is thus unlikely to exceed 9 μg.

Vitamin B_{12} deficiency is thus usually due to impaired absorption of the vitamin and not to a dietary deficiency. There is no convincing evidence of an age-related decline in B_{12} absorption despite diminution in serum B_{12} levels (Hyams, 1964; 1973), and liver stores of vitamin B_{12} are normal in 'healthy' elderly subjects (Swendseid et al., 1957). Serum B_{12} levels are subnormal in one-third of patients with nutritional megaloblastic anaemia due to folate deficiency; treatment with folic acid restores the serum B_{12} level (Mollin et al., 1962). Low serum B_{12} (radioassay) levels are also found in patients receiving massive doses of ascorbic acid (Herbert et al., 1978). Malabsorption of vitamin B_{12} may be due to gastric lesions (atrophic gastritis, pernicious anaemia, gastrectomy), intestinal lesions (gluten sensitivity, sprue, small gut infection or infestation, resection or disease, drug-induced malabsorption) or severe pancreatic disease.

Clinical Features

Although the anaemia resulting from vitamin B_{12} deficiency is technically a nutritional anaemia, the causes of that B_{12} deficiency are so rarely dietary that space will not be allocated to full descriptions of the underlying diseases. However, since pernicious anaemia is the commonest type of megaloblastic anaemia seen in the elderly, a few relevant points will be made about this disease. For a fuller account of pernicious anaemia in the elderly, see Hyams (1973); for a detailed general account, see Kass (1976).

The insidious onset leads to late diagnosis, so that the elderly may be very ill and severely anaemic before the condition is recognized. Symptoms are those of anaemia and its consequences, mental changes, and neurological changes such as peripheral neuropathy and subacute combined degeneration of the cord. On the other hand, 'latent pernicious anaemia' — vitamin B_{12} deficiency without anaemia – is also well recognized (Callender and Denborough, 1957), and MacLennan et al. (1973) found its incidence to be 5 per cent in the elderly in two Scottish communities.

Awareness of predisposing causes (e.g. past history of gastric surgery, strict vegetarianism, family history of pernicious anaemia or autoimmune disease) is the main weapon in the prevention of vitamin B_{12} deficiency states. However, it should be noted that Hughes et al. (1970) found no symptomatic benefit from vitamin B_{12} therapy in the absence of anaemia.

Oral administration of vitamin B_{12} to normal old people is unlikely to be of any value; however, it is important to vegans.

In all other instances, it will be necessary to use parenteral vitamin B_{12} injections, and these will normally need to be given regularly for life. Oral B_{12}—IF combinations may work by mouth but commonly lose their effect due to development of antibodies against the hog IF.

OTHER VITAMIN DEFICIENCIES

Data on the incidence of vitamin deficiencies in the elderly are reviewed by Brin and Bauernfeind (1978), who also indicate recommended allowance in the USA. (*See also* Chapter 3.)

Vitamin A Deficiency

Vitamin A deficiency causes anaemia in experimental animals and man, and diminution in the amount and activity of haemopoietic tissue seen in the bone marrow. The subject is reviewed by Hodges et al. (1978) who report their own studies in rats and in eight healthy middle-aged human volunteers. Anaemia developed in both studies; in man it was associated with low serum iron without a corresponding rise in TIBC. Administration of iron was of no value whilst vitamin A deficiency persisted; repletion of vitamin A led to rapid and complete haematological recovery. Although the mechanism is obscure, there is some evidence of impairment of normal erythropoiesis, production of imperfect red cells with consequent shortened life span, and haemosiderin deposition in liver and spleen.

Riboflavine Deficiency

In animals, riboflavine deficiency may produce erythroid hypoplasia of the bone marrow and a consequent aplastic anaemia. Storage of vitamin B_{12} in liver and kidney is impaired (Ellis et al., 1959). A similar picture has been noted in man. Oral symptoms and signs, such as burning and soreness of the tongue, angular stomatitis and cheilosis are often attributed to anaemia, but may be due to riboflavine deficiency alone or associated with nutritional anaemia as part of a more general malnutrition.

In treatment riboflavine is given in doses of 10–60 mg daily by the oral or parenteral route, usually together with other B-group vitamins. Response may be slow.

Old people who avoid milk, meat, fish and leafy green vegetables are particularly at risk of riboflavine deficiency and may be given prophylactic doses of 3 mg riboflavine daily, preferably with other B-complex vitamins. Such therapy led to clinical improvement in oral signs in the study reported by Dymock and Brocklehurst (1973).

Pyridoxine Deficiency

There is evidence of pyridoxine deficiency in the elderly (Ranke et al., 1960; Jacobs et al., 1968; Hoorn et al., 1975). Serum pyridoxal decreases steeply with age throughout adult life (Hamfelt, 1964; Walsh, 1966; Anderson et al., 1970; Rose et al., 1976), but because of this age-regression in serum pyridoxal concentrations, and the different assay techniques used by various authors, it is difficult to give a normal range for this parameter in elderly subjects. Values below 3 ng/ml may be subnormal; in the DHSS survey 35 per cent of subjects had such levels and 10·4 per cent had less than 2 ng/ml (Anderson et al., 1972). The cause of the age-regression in serum pyridoxal is uncertain. Hamfelt (1964) discusses the subject broadly; possibilities include defective nutrition, absorption or phosphorylation of the vitamin to its active form, increased urinary loss, and a decrease in the protein to which the vitamin is bound for transport purposes. Anderson et al. (1972) found some relationship between serum B_6 concentrations and dietary intake in the elderly, but point out that the vitamin B_6 content of food – especially during preparation – is not known with certainty. The major food sources of pyridoxine are considered to be meat and potatoes: these foods contributed approximately 26 per cent and 15–20 per cent respectively of the daily intake of pyridoxine in the DHSS survey (1972).

In animals, pyridoxine deficiency may produce a microcytic hypochromic anaemia. In human volunteers, pyridoxine deficiency is difficult to produce by dietary restriction, but has led to a hypochromic anaemia. Some patients with sideroblastic anaemia (*see* p. 109) are pyridoxine deficient: 16 of 26 patients (62 per cent) with sideroblastic anaemia studied by Anderson et al. (1970) had subnormal serum pyridoxine levels. Malabsorption states may be associated with impaired pyridoxine absorption (Baker and Sobotka, 1962; Brain and Booth, 1964) and evidence of abnormal tryptophane metabolism (Kowlessar et al., 1964). Sideroblastic anaemia may develop (Dawson et al., 1964). In such cases, correction of malabsorption (e.g. by a gluten-free diet in cases of adult coeliac disease) may correct both the pyridoxine deficiency and the sideroblastic anaemia. Other cases of sideroblastic anaemia respond to large doses of pyridoxine given over a long period; some of these will *not* have shown evidence of a specific pyridoxine deficiency before treatment. Indeed, Linman (1978) suggests that all cases of 'refractory anaemia' should be treated in this way, since a pre-leukaemic state may be the underlying cause and long-term pyridoxine therapy has sometimes decreased transfusion requirements in these patients. Sideroblastic anaemia in rheumatoid arthritis is usually associated with evidence of pyridoxine deficiency (Anderson et al., 1970), possibly due to increased requirements for pyridoxine in rheumatoid arthritis.

Doses of pyridoxine up to 150 mg per day have been given in known or suspected deficiency states; in patients with 'refractory anaemias' this treatment should be continued for 2–8 months before being discontinued if no improvement is seen. Pyridoxal-5′-phosphate treatment has been mentioned earlier in considering the sideroblastic anaemias. When pyridoxine therapy is being contemplated in the elderly without clear evidence of pyridoxine deficiency, it is worth remembering that pyridoxine will antagonize the effects of L-dopa therapy in patients with Parkinsonism.

Meat, fish, eggs, wholemeal flour, potatoes and spinach have the greatest concentrations of pyridoxine. A reasonable, balanced diet will thus prevent the development of pyridoxine deficiency unless there is malabsorption or increased requirements.

Pantothenic Acid Deficiency (Vitamin B₅)

Although reduced blood and urinary levels of pantothenic acid have been reported in the elderly (Schmidt, 1951) there is no evidence of actual deficiency of this vitamin in old age (Kirk, 1962).

In animals, experimental pantothenic acid deficiency causes hypochromic anaemia, but this is of no practical significance in man.

Niacin Deficiency (Nicotinic Acid, Vitamin B₇)

There is evidence of reduced nicotinic acid concentrations in human aortic tissue with age, from childhood to senescence (Kirk, 1962); and nicotinamide-containing enzymes are diminished in the blood of the elderly (Suvarnakich et al., 1952). Experimental niacin deficiency in animals leads to a normocytic anaemia (Marks, 1968); in man, anaemia may occur in pellagra due to deficiency of the vitamin.

Biotin Deficiency (Vitamin H)

Anaemia has been reported in experimental biotin deficiency in animals and man, but is of no practical clinical significance in the elderly.

Vitamin C Deficiency (Ascorbic Acid)

These important matters have been discussed by Exton-Smith (*see* p. 32).

1. *Roles of Vitamin C in Haemopoiesis*

Iron absorption may be facilitated by concomitant administration of vitamin C (*see above*). Iron transport may be abnormal in vitamin C deficiency states (Marks, 1968). Folic acid metabolism is impaired in vitamin C deficiency (*see above*).

A specific role for vitamin C in haemopoiesis was discussed by Goldberg (1963), Hyams and Ross (1963), Asquith et al. (1967) and Cox (1968). In a few cases, megaloblastic anaemia has responded to vitamin C as the sole therapeutic agent.

2. *Anaemia in Scurvy*

Most scorbutic patients are anaemic. The anaemia is usually normocytic or macrocytic and is normochromic. However, blood loss and iron deficiency may lead to a hypochromic microcytic anaemia. The marrow is hyperplastic and usually normoblastic, even in the presence of macrocytosis; rarely, a megaloblastic marrow is found.

Large doses of vitamin C may be given orally, from 200 to 2000 mg daily. In addition, iron, folic acid and vitamin B_{12} may be required for effective and safe treatment in certain cases.

3. *Prevention*

Dietary correction and, in selected cases, supplementary vitamin C administration, can prevent vitamin C deficiency. Particular care is needed in winter, since there is a seasonal variation in the intake of vitamin C in the diet, this being lower between October and March than between April and September (Milne et al., 1971; DHSS, 1972). Hospitals and other institutions are particularly likely to provide diets low in vitamin C, and patients and residents of such establishments should probably have routine vitamin C supplements.

Vitamin E Deficiency (Tocopherol)

This controversial substance is an anti-oxidant, the main function of which is to protect biological membranes from auto-oxidation and consequent loss of cell-integrity (Editorial, *Lancet*, 1977c). Deficiency of vitamin E causes a haemolytic anaemia in children, but this appears to be of no practical clinical significance in old age. However, in view of the possible roles of anti-oxidants in delaying the rate of ageing (Comfort, 1973) it might be wisest to keep an open mind about the possible importance of vitamin E in the elderly. Nevertheless, the recently-highlighted risk of thrombophlebitis during vitamin E therapy (Roberts, 1978) calls for caution.

Vitamin K Deficiency

Vitamin K operates at several points in the blood coagulation mechanism. Deficiency of vitamin K leads to reduction in prothrombin (Factor II) and in Factors VII, IX and X; haemorrhage may ensue. Vitamin K deficiency in the elderly (Hazell and Baloch, 1970) is not due to subnormal dietary intake of the vitamin, but may occur in malabsorption states, particularly as it is a fat-soluble vitamin. It is worth remembering that oral broad-spectrum antibiotic therapy may produce malabsorption and lead to vitamin K deficiency. Anticoagulant therapy antagonizes the effects of vitamin K by reducing hepatic synthesis of the same four coagulation factors. Diminished hepatic synthesis of these factors is also found in liver disease.

Treatment is to administer vitamin K orally or intramuscularly, according to circumstances, and to deal with any associated causative factors as far as possible. Prevention follows from the above considerations.

PROTEIN DEFICIENCY

Protein deficiency alone is said not to cause anaemia unless acting in association with other abnormalities (e.g. in cirrhosis of the liver). However, the production of erythropoietin by rats fed a protein-deficient diet is markedly decreased, and is rapidly reversible by feeding protein (Fried et al., 1957; Reissman, 1964; Anagnostou et al., 1978). It is tempting to speculate on the relationship between protein malnutrition and red-cell production in man, but evidence is lacking so far.

In view of the common occurrence of low serum albumin levels in old age (Hodkinson, 1973; Hyams, 1973; Flanagan et al., 1980) any possible relationship with the development of anaemia warrants careful investigation. Transferrin deficiency has been described (Heilmayer, 1966) and leads to a refractory hypochromic anaemia (*see above*).

A discrete normocytic normochromic anaemia has been described in association with protein—energy malnutrition in children (Fondu et al., 1978). In this anaemia, red cell survival was decreased and erythropoietin levels increased; deficiency of iron or vitamins was not the cause, and it was considered that the anaemia was distinct from that seen in chronic disorders. The possible role of selenium deficiency in the production of this anaemia is discussed, and these authors give a useful review of the literature on the subject of protein—energy malnutrition and anaemia.

REFERENCES

Anagnostou A., Schade S., Barone J. et al. (1978) *Blood* 51, 549.
Anderson B. B., Brozovic B., Mo-lin D. L. et al. (1972) In: DHSS (1972) 3 (*see* General References).
Anderson B. B., Peart M. B. and Fulford-Jones C. E. (1970) *J. Clin. Pathol.* 23, 232.

Anderson J. R., Buchanan W. W. and Goudie R. B. (1967) *Autoimmunity: Clinical and Experimental.* Springfield, Thomas.
Andrews J., Fairley A. and Barker R. (1967) *Scott. Med. J.* 12, 208.
Asquith P., Oelbaum M. H. and Dawson D. W. (1967) *Br. Med. J.* 4, 402.
Attwood E. C., Robey E., Kramer J. J. et al. (1978) *Age Ageing* 7, 46.
Baker H., Jaslow S. P. and Frank O. (1978) *J. Am. Geriatr. Soc.* 26, 218.
Baker H. and Sobotka H. (1962) *Adv. Clin. Chem.* 5, 173.
Baker S. J. (1967) *World Rev. Nutr. Diet* 8, 62.
Barry R. E., Salmon P. R., Read A. E. et al. (1971) *Gut* 12, 873.
Basu T. K. (1977) *J. Hum. Nutr.* 31, 449.
Batata M., Spray G. H., Bolton F. G. et al. (1967) *Br. Med. J.* 2, 667.
Bedford P. D. and Wollner L. (1958) *Lancet* 1, 1144.
Berg N. O., Dahlqvist A., Lindberg T. et al. (1972) *Scand. J. Haematol.* 9, 167.
Bianchi A., Chipman D. W., Dreskin A. et al. (1970) *N. Engl. J. Med.* 282, 859.
Bird T., Hall M. R. P. and Schade R. O. K. (1977) *Gerontology* 23, 309.
Björn-Rasmussen E. (1974) *Nutr. Metab.* 16, 101.
Bonnet J. D., Hagedorn A. B. and Owen C. A. (1960) *Blood* 15, 3644.
Booth J. B. and Todd G. B. (1970) *Br. J. Hosp. Med.* 4, 513.
Brain M. C. and Booth C. C. (1964) *Gut* 5, 241.
Brin M. and Bauernfeind J. C. (1978) *Postgrad. Med.* 63, 155.
Burkhardt R. (1975) (*see* General References).
Callender S. T. (1969) *Br. Med. J.* 4, 531.
Callender S. T. (1971) *Gerontol. Clin. (Basel)* 13, 44.
Callender S. T. and Denborough M. A. (1957) *Br. J. Haematol.* 3, 88.
Cartwright G. E. (1966) *Semin. Hematol.* 3, 351.
Chanarin I. (1969) *The Megaloblastic Anaemias.* Oxford, Blackwell.
Chanarin I. (1973) *Lancet* 2, 538.
Chanarin I. (1974) In: Huntsman R. G. and Jenkins G. C. (ed.), *Advanced Haematology.* London, Butterworth, p. 87.
Cleave T. L., Campbell G. D. and Painter N. S. (1969) *Diabetes, Coronary Thrombosis and the Saccharine Disease.* 2nd ed. Bristol, Wright.
Coleman D. H., Stevens A. R. and Finch C. A. (1955) *Blood* 10, 567.
Comfort A. (1973) In: Brocklehurst J. C. (ed.), *Textbook of Geriatric Medicine and Gerontology.* Edinburgh and London, Churchill Livingstone, p. 46.
Cook J. D. (1975) In: Kief H. (*see* General References), p. 272.
Cox E. V. (1968) *Vitam. Horm.* 26, 635.
Cox E. V., Meynell M. J., Gaddie R. et al. (1959) *Lancet* 2, 998.
Crosby W. H. (1978) *Am. J. Clin. Nutr.* 31, 572.
Dagg J. H., Goldberg A., Anderson J. R. et al. (1964) *Br. Med. J.* 1, 1349.
Dallman P. (1974) In: Jacobs A. and Wormwood M. (ed.), *Iron in Biochemistry and Medicine.* London, Academic, p. 43.
Das K. C. and Herbert V. (1976) *Clin. Haematol.* 5, 697.
Dawson A. M., Holdsworth C. D. and Pitcher C. S. (1964) *Gut* 5, 304.
DHSS (1969) 120 (*see* General References).
DHSS (1972) (*see* General References).
Disler P. B., Lynch S. R., Charlton R. W. et al. (1975) *Gut* 16, 193.
Dobbs R. J. and Baird I. M. (1977) *Br. Med. J.* 2, 1641.
Doniach D. and Roitt I. M. (1964) *Semin. Hematol.* 1, 313.
Dymock S. M. and Brocklehurst J. C. (1973) *Age Ageing* 2, 172.
Editorial (1976) *Br. Med. J.* 2, 71.
Editorial (1978) *Br. Med. J.* 1, 1504.
Editorial (1969) *Lancet* 2, 309.
Editorial (1976) *Lancet* 2, 836.
Editorial (1977a) *Lancet* 1, 1243.
Editorial (1977b) *Lancet* 2, 806.

Editorial (1977c) *Lancet* **2**, 1268.
Edwards F. C. and Coghill N. F. (1966) *Br. Med. J.* **2**, 1409.
Ellis L. N., Duncan B. J. and Snow I. B. (1959) *J. Nutr.* **67**, 185.
Ellwood P. C., Shinton N. K., Wilson C. I. D. et al. (1971) *Br. J. Haematol.* **21**, 557.
Ellwood P. C. and Williams G. (1970) *Practitioner* **204**, 812.
Elsborg L. (1976) *Acta Haematol.* **55**, 140.
Esposito R. (1977) *Lancet* **2**, 1132.
Evans D. M. D. (1971) *Gerontol. Clin. (Basel)* **13**, 12.
Evans D. M. D., Pathy M. S., Sanerkin N. G. et al. (1968) *Gerontol. Clin. (Basel)* **10**, 228.
Evers J. E. M. (1977) In: Fielding J. (*see* General References) p. 279.
Exton-Smith A. N. (1977) *Proc. R. Soc. Med.* **70**, 615.
Exton-Smith A. N. and Stanton B. R. (1965) *Report of an Investigation into the Dietary of Elderly Women Living Alone*. London, King Edward's Hospital Fund.
Fielding J. (1977) (*see* General References).
Flanagan R. J., Lewis R. R. and Hyams D. E. (1980) In preparation.
Fondu P., Hariga-Muller C., Mozes N. et al. (1978) *Am. J. Clin. Nutr.* **31**, 46.
Forshaw J., Moorhouse E. H. and Harwood L. (1964) *Lancet* **1**, 1004.
Franklin J. L. and Rosenberg I. G. (1973) *Gastroenterology* **64**, 517.
Freiman H. D., Tauber S. A. and Tulsky E. G. (1963) *Geriatrics* **18**, 716.
Fried W., Plzak L. F., Jacobson L. O. et al. (1957) *Proc. Soc. Exp. Biol. Med.* **94**, 237.
Girdwood R. H. (1969) *Scott. Med. J.* **14**, 296.
Goldberg A. (1963) *Q. J. Med.* **32**, 51.
Gough K. R., Read A. E., McCarthy C. F. et al. (1963) *Q. J. Med.* **32**, 243.
Green J. B. and Trowbridge A. A. (1977) *Postgrad. Med.* **61**, 149.
Hallberg L. and Högdahl A. M. (1971) *Gerontol. Clin. (Basel)* **13**, 31.
Hallberg L. and Sölvell L. (1966) *Acta Med. Scand.* Suppl. 459.
Halsted J. A., Carroll J. and Rubert S. (1959) *N. Engl. J. Med.* **260**, 575.
Hamfelt A. (1964) *Clin. Chim. Acta* **10**, 48.
Harper A. E. (1978) *Geriatrics* **33**, 73.
Hazell K. and Baloch K. H. (1970) *Gerontol. Clin. (Basel)* **12**, 10.
Heilmeyer L. (1966) *Acta Haematol.* **36**, 40.
Herbert V., Jacob E., Wong K. T. J. et al. (1978) *Am. J. Clin. Nutr.* **31**, 253.
Herbert V. and Zalusky R. (1962) *J. Clin. Invest.* **41**, 1263.
Hodges R. E., Sauberlich H. E., Canham J. E. et al. (1978) *Am. J. Clin. Nutr.* **31**, 876.
Hodkinson H. M. (1973) *Age Ageing* **2**, 157.
Hoffbrand A. V., Newcombe E. F. A. and Mollin D. L. (1966) *J. Clin. Pathol.* **19**, 17.
Holt J. M., Gear M. W. L. and Warner G. T. (1970) *Gut* **11**, 847.
Holt J. M., Mayet F. G. H., Warner G. T. et al. (1968) *Br. Med. J.* **3**, 22.
Hoorn R. K. J., Flikweert J. P. and Westerink D. (1975) *Clin. Chim. Acta* **61**, 151.
Hubbard-Ryland P. A. (1973) *Gerontol. Clin. (Basel)* **15**, 141.
Hughes D., Elwjod P. C., Shinton N. K. et al. (1970) *Br. Med. J.* **2**, 458.
Hussein S., Prieto J., O'Shea M. et al. (1975) *Br. Med. J.* **1**, 546.
Hyams D. E. (1964) *Gerontol. Clin. (Basel)* **6**, 193.
Hyams D. E. (1973) In: Brocklehurst J. C. (ed.), *Textbook of Geriatric Medicine and Gerontology*. Edinburgh and London, Churchill Livingstone.
Hyams D. E. and Ross E. J. (1963) *Br. J. Clin. Pract.* **17**, 332.
Israels M. C. G. (1975) *Mod. Geriatr.* **5**, 17.
Jacobs A. (1975) *Br. J. Haematol.* **31**, 1.
Jacobs A., Cavill I. A. J. and Hughes J. N. P. (1968) *Am. J. Clin. Nutr.* **21**, 502.
Jacobs A., Waters W. E., Campbell H. et al. (1969) *Br. J. Haematol.* **17**, 581.
Jacobs A. M. and Owen G. M. (1969) *J. Gerontol.* **24**, 95.
Joske R. A., Finckh E. S. and Wood I. J. (1955) *Q. J. Med.* **24**, 269.
Kass L. (1976) *Pernicious Anemia (Major Problems in Internal Medicine, Vol. 8)*. Philadelphia, Saunders.

Kirk J. (1962) *Vitam. Horm.* **20,** 67.

Kowlessar O. D., Haeffner L. J. and Benson G. D. (1964) *J. Clin. Invest.* **43,** 894.

Langman M. J. S. and Smithard D. J. (1977) *Br. J. Clin. Pharmacol.* **4,** 631.

Layrisse M. (1975) In: Kief H. (*see* General References) p. 25.

Layrisse M., Roche M. and Baker S. J. (1976) In: Beaton G. H. and Bengod J. M. (ed.), *Nutrition in Preventive Medicine.* Geneva, WHO, p. 55.

Lindenbaum J. and Lieber C. S. (1969) *N. Engl. J. Med.* **281,** 333.

Linman J. W. (1978) *Geriatrics* **33,** 40.

Lloyd E. L. (1971) *Gerontol. Clin. (Basel)* **13,** 246.

McCurdy P. R. and Dern R. J. (1968) *Am. J. Clin. Nutr.* **21,** 284.

McFarlane D. B., Pinkerton P. H., Dagg J. H. et al. (1967) *Br. J. Haematol.* **13,** 790.

MacLennan W. J., Andrews G. D., MacLeod C. et al. (1973) *Q. J. Med.* **42,** 1.

Manzoor M. and Runcie J. (1976) *Br. Med. J.* **1,** 1176.

Marks J. (1968) *The Vitamins in Health and Diseases: A Modern Reappraisal.* London, Churchill.

Mason D. Y. and Emerson P. M. (1973) *Br. Med. J.* **1,** 389.

Milne J. S., Lonergan M. E., Williamson J. et al. (1971) *Br. Med. J.* **4,** 383.

Mitchell T. R. and Pegrum G. D. (1971) *Gerontol. Clin. (Basel)* **13,** 296.

Mollin D. L., Waters A. H. and Harriss E. (1962) In: Heinrich H. C. (ed.), *Vitamin B_{12} and Intrinsic Factor (2nd Europ. Sympos., Hamburg, 1961).* Stuttgart, Enke, p. 737.

Myrhed M., Berglund L. and Böttiger L. E. (1977) *Acta Med. Scand.* **202,** 11.

NAS/NRC (1974) (*see* General References).

Neill D. J. (1972) In: DHSS (1972) 3 (*see* General References).

Nordin B. E. C., Williamson A. R., Marshall D. H. et al. (1976) *Calc. Tiss. Res.* **21,** Suppl., 442.

Noronha J. M. and Silverman M. (1962) In: Heinrich H. C. (ed.), *Vitamin B_{12} und Intrinsic Factor (2nd Europ. Sympos., Hamburg, 1961).* Stuttgart, Enke, p. 728.

Olsson K. S. (1977) In: Fielding J. (*see* General References) p. 392.

Passmore R., Nicol B. M. and Rao M. N. (1974) *Handbook on Human Nutritional Requirements.* Geneva, WHO.

Perry J., Lumb M. and Laundy M. (1976) *Br. J. Haematol.* **32,** 243.

Pincus J. H., Reynolds E. H. and Glaser G. H. (1972) *J. Am. Med. Assoc.* **221,** 496.

Pitney W. R. and Onesti P. (1961) *Aust. J. Exp. Biol. Med. Sci.* **39,** 1.

Polland W. S. (1933) *Arch. Intern. Med.* **51,** 903.

Powell D. B. and Thomas J. H. (1969) *Gerontol. Clin. (Basel)* **11,** 36.

Powell D. E. B., Thomas J. H. and Mills P. (1968) *Gerontol. Clin. (Basel)* **10,** 21.

Pryce J. D. (1960) *Lancet* **333.**

Ranke E., Tauber S. A., Horonick A. et al. (1960) *J. Gerontol.* **15,** 41.

Raper C. F. L. and Choudhury M. (1978) *J. Clin. Pathol.* **31,** 44.

Read A. E., Gough K. R., Pardoe J. L. et al. (1965) *Br. Med. J.* **2,** 843.

Reissman K. R. (1964) *Blood* **23,** 146.

Reynolds E. H. (1976a) *Lancet* **2,** 822.

Reynolds E. H. (1976b) *Clin. Haematol.* **5,** 661.

Roberts H. J. (1978) *Lancet* **1,** 49.

Rose C. S., György P., Butler M. et al. (1976) *Am. J. Clin. Nutr.* **29,** 847.

Rosenberg I. H. (1976) *Clin. Haematol.* **5,** 589.

Schmidt V. (1951) *J. Gerontol.* **6,** 132.

Schneider R. E. and Beeley L. (1977) *Br. Med. J.* **2,** 1638.

Scott J. T., Porter I. H., Lewis S. M. et al. (1961) *Q. J. Med.* **30,** 167.

Shaw D. M. (1971) In: Arnstein H. R. V. and Wrighton R. J. (ed.), *The Cobalamins: A Glaxo Symposium.* Edinburgh and London, Churchill Livingstone, p. 109.

Shin Y. S., Buehring K. U. and Stokstad E. L. R. (1975) *Mol. Cell. Biochem.* **9,** 97.

Sneath P., Chanarin I., Hodgkinson H. M. et al. (1973) *Age Ageing* **2,** 177.

Stanton B. R. and Exton-Smith A. N. (1970) *A Longitudinal Study of the Dietary of Elderly Women.* London, King Edward's Hospital Fund.

Stewart J. S., Roberts P. D. and Hoffbrand A. V. (1970) *Lancet* **2**, 542.

Strachan R. W. and Henderson J. G. (1967) *Q. J. Med.* **36**, 189.

Strauss R. G. (1978) *Am. J. Clin. Nutr.* **31**, 660.

Sundin T. (1977) In: Fielding J. (*see* General References), pp. 222 and 392.

Suvarnakich K., Mann G. V. and Stare F. J. (1952) *J. Nutr.* **47**, 105.

Swendseid M. E., Gasster M. and Halsted J. A. (1954) *Proc. Soc. Exp. Biol. Med.* **86**, 834.

Swendseid M. E., Hvollboll E., Schick G. et al. (1957) *Blood* **12**, 24.

Thomas J. H. (1971) *Gerontol. Clin. (Basel)* **13**, 52.

Thomas J. H. and Powell D. E. B. (1971) *Blood Disorders in the Elderly.* Bristol, Wright.

Trump B. F., Barrett L. A., Valigorsky J. M. et al. (1975) In: Kief H. (*see* General References) p. 251.

Turnbull A. (1971) *Br. J. Hosp. Med.* **6**, 537.

Vancini B., Lanfranchi G. A., Puddu P. et al. (1967) *Arch. Pathol. Clin. Med.* **43**, 175.

Vanzant F. R., Alvarez W. C., Eusterman G. B. et al. (1932) *Arch. Intern. Med.* **49**, 345.

Vilter R. W. (1964) *Medicine (Baltimore)* **43**, 727.

Viteri F. E., Alvarado J., Luthringer D. G. et al. (1968) *Vitam. Horm.* **26**, 573.

Walder A. I. (1968) *Surgery* **64**, 175.

Walsh M. P. (1966) *Am. J. Clin. Pathol.* **46**, 282.

Wangel A. G., Callender S. T., Spray G. H. et al. (1968) *Br. J. Haematol.* **14**, 161.

Wapnick A. A., Lynch S. R., Charlton R. W. et al. (1969) *Br. J. Haematol.* **17**, 563.

Webster S. G. P. and Leeming J. T. (1975) *Age Ageing* **4**, 168.

Weeks B. and Krasilnikoff P. A. (1972) *Acta Med. Scand.* **192**, 149.

WHO (1968) *Nutritional Anaemias. WHO Techn. Rep. Ser. No. 405.* Geneva, WHO.

WHO (1970) *Requirements of Ascorbic Acid, Vitamin D, Vitamin B_{12}, Folate and Iron. WHO Techn. Rep. Ser. No. 452.* Geneva, WHO.

WHO (1972) *Nutritional Anaemias. WHO Techn. Rep. Ser. No. 503.* Geneva, WHO.

WHO (1975) *Control of Nutritional Anaemia with Special Reference to Iron Deficiency. WHO Techn. Rep. Ser. No. 580.* Geneva, WHO.

Wickramasinghe S. N. and Longland J. E. (1974) *Br. Med. J.* **3**, 148.

Wintrobe M. M. (1967) *Clinical Haematology,* 6th ed. Philadelphia, Lea and Febiger.

Witts L. J. (1966) *The Stomach and Anaemia.* London, Athlone, p. 30.

Witts L. J. (1969) *Hypochromic Anaemia.* London, Heinemann.

Wright W. B. (1967) *Gerontol. Clin. (Basel)* **9**, 107.

Wu A., Chanarin I. and Levi A. J. (1974) *Lancet* **1**, 829.

Wu A., Chanarin I., Slavin G. et al. (1975) *Br. J. Haematol.* **29**, 469.

Zittoun J., Marquet J. and Zittoun R. (1978) *Blood* **51**, 119.

11. CALCIUM METABOLISM AND BONE
B. E. C. Nordin

It is common knowledge that fracture rates rise with age, more particularly in women, and that the principal skeletal sites affected are the distal fore-arm, vertebrae and proximal femur. Although some element of trauma is involved in most of these fractures, the increased liability to falls in the elderly is certainly not sufficient to account for the rise in fracture rate, and it is clear that age-related loss of bone is a major contributory factor. The present chapter will therefore examine the changes in bone mass and bone quality which accompany ageing and review available evidence regarding the hormonal and nutritional factors involved in these processes.

LOSS OF BONE WITH AGE
The dry weight of the skeleton represents about 8 per cent of body weight in young healthy adults (Nordin, 1976), 80 per cent of it being cortical or compact bone and 20 per cent trabecular bone (Trotter et al., 1960). In absolute terms, most loss of tissue with age comes from cortical bone, but in proportional terms it is the trabecular bone which is most severely affected.

Cortical Bone Loss
The loss of cortical bone with age is most easily monitored by means of cortical width measurements on standard radiographs. Such measurements have been performed on the femur, tibia, clavicle, radius and other bones (Horsman, 1976), but the site most commonly chosen is the mid-point of the second metacarpal of the right hand (Barnett and Nordin, 1960). Cortical width at this site declines by about 1 per cent per annum from the age of 50 in women, and somewhat more slowly and starting later in men. However, cross-sectional area is in fact a better measure of tubular bone mass than cortical width and it is therefore customary to measure meta-carpal medullary and total width, calculate medullary and total area on the assumption that the bone is cylindrical and derive a value for cross-sectional cortical area (CA), which declines at about 0·8 per cent per annum in women and about 0·2 per cent in men. CA varies widely between young normal individuals (coefficient of variation about 13 per cent) and this variance can be substantially reduced by relating CA to the total cross-sectional area of the bone (TA) and expressing the result as the CA/TA ratio (Garn, 1970) which has a coefficient of variation of about

6 per cent in young normal people. An alternative approach is to relate cortical width to metacarpal surface area as suggested by Exton-Smith et al. (1969).

The changes in the metacarpal which accompany ageing are illustrated in *Fig.* 11.1 and arise from endosteal resorption, which causes expansion of the medullary cavity, partially offset by apposition of bone on the periosteal surface. Intracortical resorption also contributes some loss of bone which is not detected by X-ray morphometry. The two latter processes

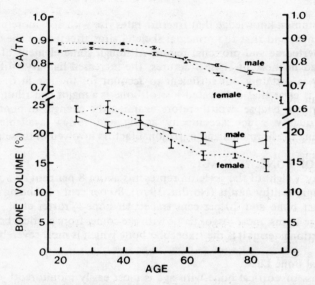

Fig. 11.1. Metacarpal CA/TA values as a function of age in normal men and women (*above*) and iliac crest trabecular bone volumes (*below*). (Metacarpal data from Garn, 1970. Iliac crest data from Meunier et al., 1973 and Gallagher et al., 1973a.)

are of minor significance in the metacarpal but of considerable importance in the femur where subperiosteal apposition of bone more than offsets endosteal resorption (Smith and Walker, 1964) and loss of femoral cortical tissue is entirely accounted for by intracortical resorption (Sissons et al., 1967).

There is little doubt that the onset of cortical bone loss in women is related to the menopause rather than to age as such. This can be demonstrated by examining data from oophorectomized women, in whom the relation between age and bone status is very weak but the correlation between bone status and years since menopause is highly significant (Gallagher et al., 1973b). It is of interest in this connection to note that sequential radiographic morphometry in post-menopausal women shows that bone loss proceeds more rapidly in the first three years after the menopause than it does subsequently. This is particularly clear after oophorectomy (Horsman et al. 1977b) but also applies to normal post-menopausal women, although the change in rate of bone loss is less clear in this group because the exact date of the menopause is more difficult to define in normal than oophorectomized women.

Trabecular Bone Loss

Trabecular bone loss has been studied most extensively in the vertebrae and the iliac crest. In post-mortem studies on vertebrae, Arnold (1973) reported a 50 per cent loss of vertebral tissue between youth and old age in both sexes. Rather comparable results have been reported by Sissons et al. (1967) in the iliac crest. The iliac crest data of Meunier et al. (1973) and Aaron (1976) show that women start with a slightly higher mean bone volume than men but lose bone more rapidly in middle life and have less bone than men in old age (*Fig.* 11.1). The mean trabecular bone volume in men and women below 50 is 22 per cent, in men over 60 it is 19 per cent and in women over 60 it is 16 per cent. Thus men lose 17 per cent of their initial trabecular bone mass and women 29 per cent, the difference between them being presumably attributable to the menopause. It should be noted that whereas cortical bone loss continues in both sexes to the end of life, trabecular bone loss seems to slow down or cease after the age of 60 (*Fig.* 11.1).

AGE-RELATED FRACTURES

Lower Forearm Fractures

There is a sharp rise in the incidence of lower forearm fractures in women from about the age of 50 which reaches a plateau of about 40 cases per 10 000 per annum in women over 65. The cumulative prevalence reaches about 5 per cent of women by age 60 and 14 per cent by age 80 (*Fig.* 11.2). There is a much slower rise in the lower forearm fracture rate in men. In our series of 107 unselected female Colles' fracture cases, 103 were post-menopausal and only 4 pre-menopausal (Gallagher and Nordin, 1974). Since the distal radius, where this fracture occurs, is composed largely of trabecular bone, and since the rise in Colles' fracture incidence plateaus at about age 65, like the trabecular bone loss in the iliac crest (*Fig.* 11.1), it seems reasonable to conclude that this fracture is the result of trabecular bone loss in the distal forearm. What is perhaps surprising is that, although the mean age of these fracture cases (in our series) is 65 years and the mean time elapsed since the menopause is 12 years, many of these patients sustain their fractures within a very short time of the menopause when they can only have lost a very small fraction of their trabecular bone. It must be remembered, however, that this fracture always results from considerable trauma (a fall on the outstretched arm) and the explanation may be that the 'safety margin' in the distal forearm is so small that a very

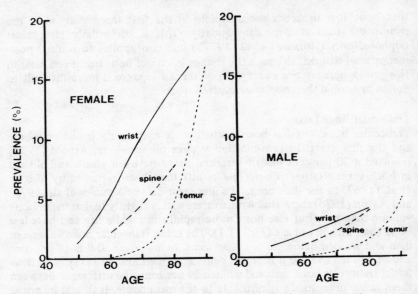

Fig. 11.2. Cumulative prevalences of wrist, spine and proximal femur fractures in men and women as a function of age. (Marshall and Nordin.)

slight loss of bone is sufficient to increase the fracture risk. On the hypothesis of Newton-John and Morgan (1970), it would be expected that distal forearm trabecular bone mass in Colles' fracture cases would be more than one standard deviation below the young normal mean, and this is largely borne out by forearm densitometry measurements on Colles' fracture cases (*Fig.* 11.3). Unfortunately, for technical reasons, forearm densitometry has to be performed at a site proximal to the actual fracture site and so a substantial proportion of the photon absorption is attributable to cortical rather than trabecular bone. This may explain why some of the values in the fracture cases fall well within the young normal range, but it may also be that loss of bone *in the individual* is more important than the relative bone status between individuals.

Vertebral Compression Fractures

Vertebral compression fractures constitute the syndrome to which the term 'osteoporosis' is commonly applied, and this terminology tends to be validated by the low iliac crest bone volumes reported in these cases by Meunier et al. (1973) and Gallagher et al. (1973a).

The incidence and prevalence of the crush fracture syndrome have not been satisfactorily established. It is, of course, a recognized complication of hyperthyroidism, of Cushing's syndrome and of corticosteroid therapy ('secondary osteoporosis'), but it is also relatively common in the elderly

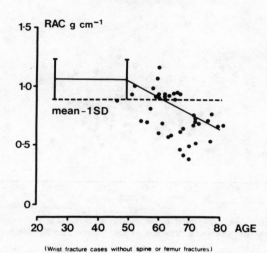

MINERAL CONTENT OF RADIUS IN
COLLES' FRACTURE CASES
(contralateral arm)

Fig. 11.3. Radial ash content, determined by photon absorptiometry, in female wrist fracture cases. The solid line indicates the mean normal value and the interrupted line the normal mean minus one standard deviation. (Horsman and Nordin.)

population at large ('primary osteoporosis'). Smith and Rizek (1966) reported a prevalence of 26 per cent in institutionalized women (average age 85) and 5 per cent in institutionalized men (average age 63). Such estimates are critically dependent upon whether *wedged* vertebrae are accepted as indicators of osteoporosis or whether the diagnosis is confined to cases where there is true vertebral *compression*. We estimate that 8 per cent of women and perhaps 4 per cent of men develop true vertebral compression by age 80 (*Fig.* 11.2).

There is little doubt that vertebral compression is generally associated with a diminished vertebral trabecular bone volume. Arnold (1973) found that vertebral compression tended to be associated with vertebral ash values below 0·07 g/ml. Reference to the compressive strength studies of Weaver and Chalmers (1966) shows that vertebral mass values in this range would be associated with failure strengths below about 700 kPa (100 lb/sq in) compared with a strength of about 5000 kPa (700 lb/sq in) in young adults.

This diminished trabecular bone volume is reflected in the iliac crest, where the bone volume is generally below 6 per cent in crush fracture cases of both sexes compared with the normal mean value in young adults

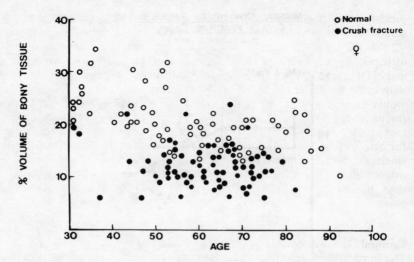

Fig. 11.4. Iliac crest trabecular bone volume in normal females (acute deaths) and crush fracture cases as a function of age. (Aaron and Nordin.)

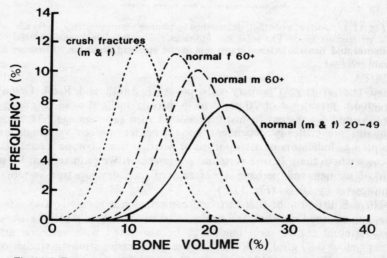

Fig. 11.5. Frequency distributions of trabecular bone volume in young normal individuals, normal men and women over 60 and crush fracture cases. (Derived from data in *Figs.* 11.1. and 11.4.)

of 22 per cent (*Fig.* 11.4). The frequency distribution curves of iliac crest bone volume in normal young adults, normal elderly men and women and crush fracture cases of both sexes is shown in *Fig.* 11.5. It is clear that a precise definition of histological 'osteoporosis' is difficult and must be somewhat arbitrary, but the lower limit of the young normal range (mean −2 S.D.) is 16 per cent and if values of 15 per cent or less are classified as osteoporotic, then 13 per cent of normal young adults, 50 per cent of normal old women, 20 per cent of normal old men and 80 per cent of patients with crush fractures would have histological osteoporosis. The implication would be that although 50 per cent of old women are at risk of crush fractures only one-sixth of these (8 per cent) actually develop them (see above). Similarly, although 20 per cent of normal old men are at risk for osteoporosis, only about one-fifth (4 per cent) actually develop crush fractures. Thus the main reason why fewer men than women develop osteoporosis is simply that the normal bone volume in old men is greater than in old women, presumably because men do not have a menopause.

Femoral Neck Fractures

The femoral neck fracture rate rises in both sexes from the seventh decade onwards and continues to rise to the end of life, more rapidly in women than in men (Knowelden et al., 1964). The cumulative prevalence reaches 5 in women by age 80 and 16 by age 90, the corresponding figures in men being 1·5 and 5 respectively (Fig. 11.2).

Cortical bone status in femoral neck fracture cases below 65 is essentially normal and most of these fractures are traumatic (Fig. 11.6). Over age 65, fracture cases tend to have less bone than normal for their age with a mean CA/TA equivalent to the normal mean at age 80. Expressed in another way, the actual CA/TA in most fracture cases over 65 is more than two standard deviations below the young normal mean (Fig. 11.6). This is compatible with the concept of Newton-John and Morgan (1970) that fracture incidence rises with age because the number of individuals with bone mass below the lower young normal limit, and so at risk for fracture, increases with age. However, they imply that all subjects lose bone at the same rate and that those who enter the fracture risk zone first are simply those who reach middle life with the least bone. It seems more likely that the rate of bone loss rather than the initial bone status is the main determinant of bone status in the elderly — but perhaps both factors are involved.

Trabecular bone status in femoral neck fracture cases is more complex. In our series, the mean iliac crest bone volumes are distributed throughout the 'normal' range for elderly subjects and include a considerable proportion of both high and low values (Fig. 11.7). Only about 30 per cent of our females (61/189) and 15 per cent of our males (5/31) have biopsy volumes below 16 per cent denoting 'osteoporosis' as defined above (Table 11.1) which is no higher than the expected proportion in the normal population (see above).

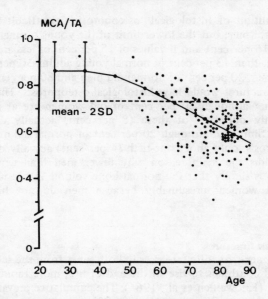

Fig. 11.6. Metacarpal CA/TA ratios in female femoral neck fracture cases. The solid line indicates the normal mean and the interrupted line denotes the normal mean minus two standard deviations. (Horsman and Nordin.)

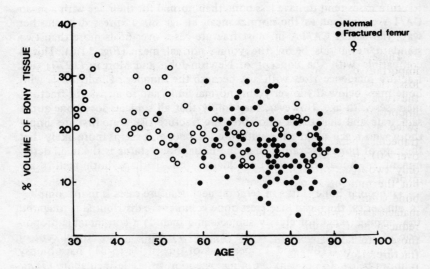

Fig. 11.7. Iliac crest trabecular bone volumes in female fractured femur cases and controls as a function of age. (Aaron, Gallagher and Nordin.)

Table 11.1. Femoral neck fracture cases classified into normal, osteoporotic and osteomalacic on the basis of iliac crest biopsies

| | | Females (189) Osteomalacia | | |
		Absent	Present	Total
	Absent	87	41	128
OSTEOPOROSIS	Present	52	9	61
	Total	139	50	189

| | | Males (31) Osteomalacia | | |
		Absent	Present	Total
	Absent	19	7	26
OSTEOPOROSIS	Present	5	0	5
	Total	24	7	31

Table 11.2 Relation between iliac crest bone volume and fracture type in female cases

| | Fracture type | |
	Pertrochanteric	Other
Bone > 15%	14	42
Volume ≤ 15%	39	26

Chi-square 14·5: $P > 0·0005$

These data might suggest that cortical bone loss is generally a more important determinant of femoral neck fracture than is trabecular bone loss. However, analysis of the trabecular bone volume data in relation to the type of femoral fracture suggests that trabecular bone loss makes an important contribution to the pertrochanteric fracture, which is about twice as common as the transcervical fracture. As *Table* 11.2 shows, trabecular bone volumes below 16 per cent (the normal mean in women over 60) are found in nearly four-fifths of pertrochanteric fractures and only two-fifths of cervical fractures in women. Our male data are similar but the numbers much smaller. This relation between reduced trabecular bone volume and pertrochanteric fracture also applies *within* the 42 osteo-malacia cases, which are included in *Table* 11.2. Thus osteomalacics with reduced bone volume are more liable to the pertrochanteric fracture and those with normal or high bone volume more liable to the transcervical fracture. However, it is impossible to say from these data whether low trabecular volume determines the fracture itself or simply the site of the fracture.

Iliac crest biopsies have also shown that osteomalacia is more common in femoral neck fractures than has been thought (Aaron et al., 1974a). In a substantial proportion of iliac crest biopsies from femoral neck fracture cases, there is an increased percentage of osteoid-covered surfaces and a reduced percentage of calcification fronts. In our series, such evidence of osteomalacia was found in 50 of 189 biopsies from female femoral neck fractures and 7 of 31 biopsies from males (*Table* 11.1). This is a much higher incidence of osteomalacia than obtains in our control (post-mortem) material in which we have found increased osteoid and/or reduced calcification fronts in only 3 of 24 men and 4 of 36 women over 60. Moreover, the osteomalacia in femoral neck fractures was seasonal (Aaron et al., 1974b); the proportion of cases with decreased calcification fronts or increased osteoid-covered surfaces rose from about 15 per cent of the biopsies in the late summer to 40 per cent in the spring (*Fig.* 11.8) which

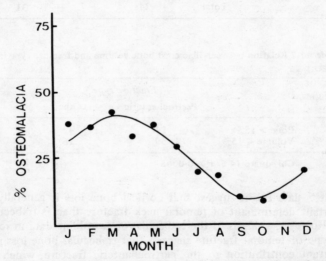

Fig. 11.8. Percentage of osteomalacic iliac crest biopsies in femoral neck fracture cases arranged by months of the year. (Aaron, Gallagher and Nordin.)

suggests that these abnormalities are genuine manifestations of vitamin D deficiency (*see below*). In addition, vitamin D therapy has been shown to correct both the abnormal forming surfaces and the abnormal calcification fronts (*Fig.* 11.9) though, interestingly enough, this is always associated with a loss of trabecular bone (*Fig.* 11.10).

Rather similar data on the incidence of osteomalacia in femoral neck fracture cases have been reported by Jenkins et al. (1973), O'Driscoll (1973) and Faccini et al. (1976) whereas Hodkinson (1971) found virtually no osteomalacia in his femoral neck fracture series. However, Hodkinson used as his criterion of osteomalacia the thickness of osteoid seams rather

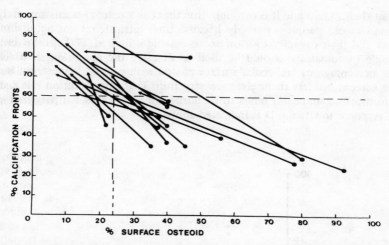

Fig. 11.9. Percent surface osteoid and percent calcification fronts in femoral neck fracture cases before and after vitamin D therapy. (Aaron, Gallagher and Nordin.)

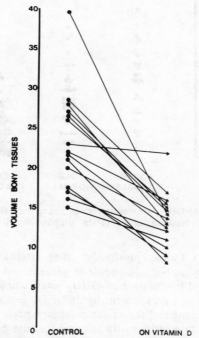

Fig. 11.10. Iliac crest trabecular bone volume in femoral neck fracture cases before and after vitamin D therapy. (Aaron, Gallagher and Nordin.)

than their extent and it is certainly true that thick osteoid seams are rarely found in old people – possibly because their intrinsic rate of bone turnover and their capacity to form excess osteoid is limited. Perhaps the term 'senile osteomalacia' should be used to describe the condition in which the percentage of trabecular surface coated with osteoid is increased but the osteoid borders themselves are very thin. That this condition is in fact a form of osteomalacia tends to be borne out by its seasonal pattern and its response to vitamin D as indicated above.

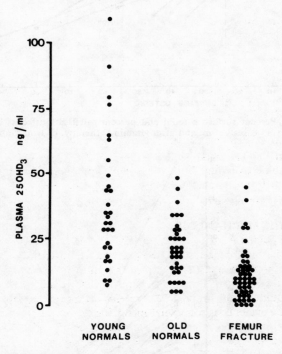

Fig. 11.11. Plasma 25-OHD$_3$ concentrations in young normals, elderly normals and femoral neck fracture cases. (Data supplied by Baker, Morris and Peacock.)

Exton-Smith (1971) has previously called attention to evidence of vitamin D deficiency among old people in general, and Stamp and Round (1974) have reported low plasma 25-OHD$_3$ levels among the elderly. This has been confirmed in Leeds where the 25-OHD$_3$ levels in old people are lower than in the young and the values in femoral neck fracture cases even lower (*Fig.* 11.11). In a series of 45 femoral fracture cases in which both biopsies and 25-OHD$_3$ levels were obtained, there was a clear association between histological osteomalacia and low plasma vitamin D levels (*Table*

11.3). Although it is possible (though unusual) to find plasma 25-OHD$_3$ levels below 10 ng/ml in old people without osteomalacia, it is very exceptional to find osteomalacia in association with a plasma level over 10 ng/ml.

There are probably two factors involved in the poor vitamin D status of elderly persons in general and femoral neck fracture cases in particular — exposure and nutrition. Solar irradiation in the UK is at best marginal (*see* Chapter 10) and probably inadequate to maintain vitamin D status in elderly people who are less exposed than the young to such sunlight as is

Table 11.3. Relation between plasma 25-OHD$_3$ level and histological osteomalacia in 45 cases of femoral neck fracture (Aaron et al.)

	Osteomalacia	
	Absent	Present
Plasma 25-OHD$_3$ < 10	9	11
(ng/ml) ⩾ 10	22	3

Chi-square 7·7: $P > 0.01$

available. In addition, the reduced appetite and reduced income of the elderly combine to reduce both the quality and quantity of their diet and prevent them from making up from dietary sources the vitamin D they are not deriving from sunlight.

PATHOGENIC MECHANISMS
Histological Evidence
It is clear that age-related bone loss must be associated with a decline in the rate of bone formation, a rise in the rate of bone resorption or a combination of the two. It might be thought that histological examination of bone would demonstrate clearly which of these was the dominant factor but the evidence is somewhat inconclusive.

As far as resorption is concerned, Meunier et al. (1973) reported no change in percentage resorption surfaces with age in women but Melsen et al. (1978) showed a small rise in resorption in women over 50. The Leeds data are shown in *Fig.* 11.12. In post-mortem material from women below 50, the percentage of resorption surfaces is almost invariably below 6 per cent whereas in women over 50 values of up to 12 per cent or even more are seen. The difference between these two groups is highly significant. However, percent resorption is no higher in our osteoporotic than non-osteoporotic cases.

In males, Meunier et al. (1973) again report no increase in bone resorption with age and the Leeds data are in agreement with this observation (*Fig.* 11.12) but there is a tendency for resorption to be raised in our male osteoporotics.

As far as forming surfaces are concerned, Meunier et al. (1973) report

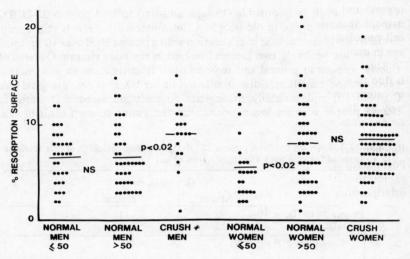

Fig. 11.12. Percent resorption surfaces in iliac crest samples from young, old and osteoporotic men and women. (Aaron.)

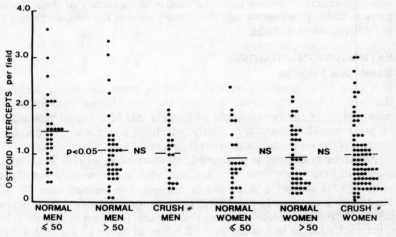

Fig. 11.13. Osteoid intercepts per field in young, old and osteoporotic men and women. (Aaron.)

no change in osteoid volume with age in women but a decline in the cell population of the marrow, which they take to indicate a reduction in bone formation rate expressed as the mean number of forming surfaces per histological field. The Leeds data are shown in *Fig.* 11.13. There is no difference in forming surfaces between young and old women or between normal and osteoporotic women. In men, Meunier et al. report no fall in osteoid volume with age but some decline in the volume of the marrow cell population. The Leeds data suggest a decline in bone formation with age in men but no difference between normal and osteoporotic men.

Thus our histological evidence suggests that post-menopausal bone loss is due to a rise in bone resorption, but does not explain the excessive loss in osteoporosis. Our male data suggest that age-related bone loss in men may be due to reduced bone formation but that osteoporosis in men may be due to increased bone resorption.

Biochemical Evidence

Post-menopausal women have a significantly higher urinary hydroxyproline excretion than pre-menopausal women, and the excretion is even higher in osteoporotic women (*Fig.* 11.14). Thus the biochemistry suggests that

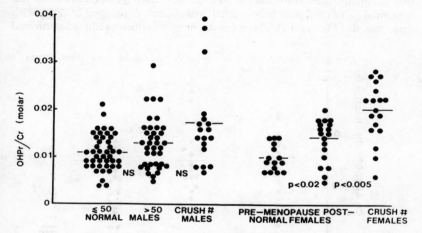

Fig. 11.14. Fasting urinary hydroxyproline/creatinine ratios in young, old and osteoporotic men and women. (The normal and osteoporotic post-menopausal women are matched for years since menopause.)

post-menopausal osteopenia is associated with an increase in bone resorption rate and post-menopausal osteoporosis with an even greater rate of bone resorption. There is some rise in urinary hydroxyproline with age in men, but it is not significant, nor is the hydroxyproline excretion significantly higher in osteoporotic than normal elderly men, but it is significantly higher than in normal young men (*Fig.* 11.14). However, the scatter of the data is very great and suggests that male osteoporosis is not a single entity.

The increased bone resorption in post-menopausal women can be attributed to an alteration in the sensitivity of bone to parathyroid hormone in the absence of oestrogens, as originally suggested by Heaney (1965) and

Jasani et al. (1965). An alternative explanation is provided by Klotz et al. (1975) and Hillyard et al. (1978) who have reported that plasma calcitonin levels are lower in women than in men and that they can be raised by oestrogen administration and implied that post-menopausal bone resorption may be due to a fall in calcitonin levels.

Whatever the cause the increase in bone resorption at the menopause raises the plasma and urine calcium (Gallagher et al., 1972) and this probably explains the somewhat reduced plasma parathyroid hormone levels (Riggs et al., 1973) and $1,25(OH)_2 D_3$ levels (Gallagher et al., 1976) in post-menopausal osteoporosis. In fact, it may be that this partial suppression of parathyroid and 1,25 secretion is the key to post-menopausal osteoporosis, the levels being sufficient to maintain bone resorption but not to maintain calcium absorption (Gallagher et al., 1973).

Thus post-menopausal osteoporosis appears to result from a combination of calcium malabsorption and oestrogen deficiency. Calcium absorption is normal in normal post-menopausal women but is reduced in those with osteoporosis (*Fig.* 11.15). Plasma oestrone is, of course, reduced in normal

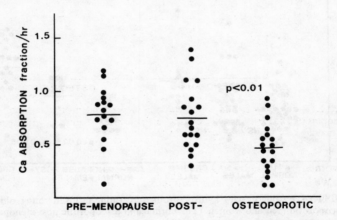

*Fig.*11.15. Radiocalcium absorption in pre-menopausal, post-menopausal and osteoporotic women. (The normal and osteoporotic post-menopausal women are matched for years since menopause.)

post-menopausal women but is even lower in those with osteoporosis (*Fig.* 11.16) (Marshall et al., 1977). Whether these are related or independent abnormalities is still not entirely clear; perhaps a vicious cycle is set up in which increased bone resorption suppresses calcium absorption (as suggested above) and malabsorption of calcium perpetuates the bone resorption (Nordin et al., 1976).

The cause of the declining bone formation rate with age in men is not known, but it is associated with and may be attributable to the declining secretion of testicular testosterone which starts in the third decade and continues to the end of life, producing a steady decline in the plasma testosterone level (Baker et al., 1976). However, the plasma testosterone is not significantly reduced in most cases of male osteoporosis, nor is malabsorption of calcium such a common finding as in the female cases. Conceivably, low dietary calcium is a more important risk factor in men

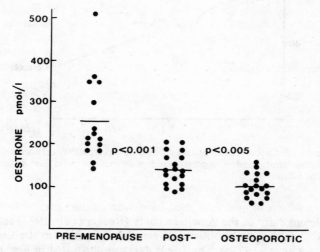

Fig. 11.16. Plasma oestrone concentrations in pre- and post-menopausal and osteoporotic women. (The normal and osteoporotic post-menopausal women are matched for years since menopause.)

than women, and might explain the osteoporosis of alcoholism (Saville, 1965). We have observed that a number of our male cases have been taking anticonvulsant therapy but the way in which this might predispose to osteoporosis is not clear.

PREVENTION AND TREATMENT
Post-menopausal Osteopenia
Bone loss in normal post-menopausal women can be prevented with oestrogen therapy and delayed if not entirely prevented by calcium supplements. The oestrogen effect has been demonstrated with mestranol (Lindsay et al., 1976), ethinyloestradiol (Horsman et al., 1977a) and Premarin (Recker et al., 1977). The Leeds data are illustrated in *Fig.* 11.17 and show no loss of metacarpal bone in over 60 patient years on oestrogen. The regime used was ethinyloestradiol 25–50 μg daily for 3 weeks out of 4, but we now know that bone resorption can be controlled by doses in the range 15–25 μg daily.

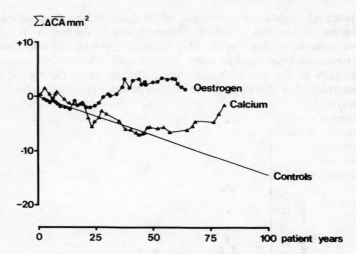

Fig. 11.17. Cusum plots of changes in mean metacarpal cortical area in oestrogen and calcium-treated post-menopausal women. The solid line indicates the control data.

The calcium supplements used have been calcium carbonate to provide 1 g calcium daily in the American study (Recker et al., 1977) and calcium Sandoz 2 tablets daily 800 mg of elemental calcium) in the Leeds study (Horsman et al., 1977a). The Leeds data are illustrated in *Fig.* 11.17 and show that bone loss has been substantially delayed if not totally prevented in 80 patient years on calcium supplements.

Post-menopausal Osteoporosis

A variety of treatments have been recommended for established post-menopausal osteoporosis. They include oestrogens, fluoride, vitamin D, calcium supplements and anabolic steroids.

Jowsey et al. (1972) recommend a combination of sodium fluoride 50 mg daily, vitamin D 50 000 units twice weekly and calcium supplements, and have reported an increase in bone volume on iliac crest biopsy on this therapy. However, this increase in bone volume is largely attributable to the development of non-calcifiable osteoid of the type seen in fluorosis and there is no satisfactory evidence that this in itself yields any clinical benefit to the patients. Any other benefit from this treatment could of course be due to the vitamin D and calcium (*see below*).

As far as anabolic steroids are concerned, Chesnut et al. (1976) have made repeated measurements of total body calcium in osteoporotic patients treated with Methandrostenolone and untreated controls and have reported a significant benefit from this compound. We know of no convincing data on the value of any other anabolic steroids in osteoporosis.

In Leeds, six different therapies for post-menopausal osteoporosis have been assessed. Initially, patients with normal calcium absorption were given calcium supplements to provide 800–1200 mg of extra calcium daily and patients with malabsorption of calcium were given 10 000–50 000 units daily of vitamin D, some with and some without calcium supplements. More recently, patients have been given 1α-OHD$_3$ (or $1,25(OH)_2D_3$) in doses of $1–2$ μg daily, or hormones or a combination of the two. The hormone preparation has generally been ethinyloestradiol 25 μg per day cyclically but where oestrogens were contraindicated we have used Nor-ethisterone 5 mg daily. Apart from the original selection of normal absorbers for simple calcium therapy, the allocation of the patients to the treatment groups has been entirely arbitrary.

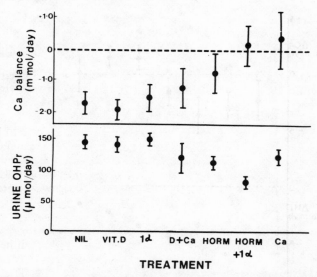

Fig. 11.18. Mean calcium balances and urine hydroxyproline ($\pm$ s.e.) in post-menopausal osteoporotic women untreated and on 6 different therapies.

The effect of these therapies has been assessed by short-term and long-term observations. The short-term observations have included the measurement of calcium balance and urinary hydroxyproline, the object being of course to reduce bone resorption and improve calcium balance. Long-term observations include the sequential measurement of mean metacarpal cortical area and the assessment of vertebral fracture progression by the measurement of height.

As far as the short-term observations are concerned, the calcium balance and urinary hydroxyproline in untreated cases of post-menopausal osteoporosis and in subgroups of the same patients on six different therapies are illustrated in *Fig.* 11.18. The calcium balance in the untreated state was significantly negative. The only treatment which produced a positive balance was the combination of 1α-OHD$_3$ with hormones, but on hormone therapy alone and calcium therapy alone the negative calcium balances were very small. The least satisfactory, most negative calcium balances were seen in the groups on vitamin D, 1α-OHD$_3$ and vitamin D plus calcium. Conversely, the lowest mean urinary hydroxyproline (indicating the lowest bone resorption) was seen in the group on hormones plus 1α-OHD$_3$ and the next lowest in the group on hormones alone. The highest urinary hydroxyprolines were seen in the patients on vitamin D and 1α-OHD$_3$.

The long-term data are illustrated in *Fig.* 11.19. There was a gain in metacarpal cortical area in the groups on hormones and hormones plus

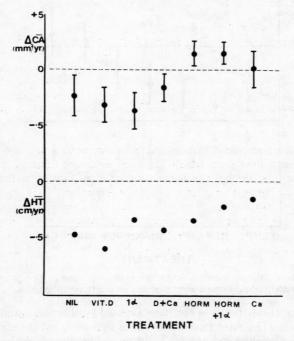

Fig. 11.19. Mean rates of change (± s.e.) in mean metacarpal cortical area in post-menopausal osteoporotic women, untreated and on 6 different therapies (*above*) and the corresponding changes in height (*below*).

1α-OHD$_3$, no significant change in mean cortical area in the group on calcium, a significant loss of bone in the untreated cases but an even greater loss in the groups on vitamin D and 1α-OHD$_3$; the vitamin D plus calcium group occupied an intermediate position. The changes in standing height were compatible with these data. The greatest loss of height occurred in the vitamin D-treated group and the least loss of height in the groups on calcium and on hormones plus 1α-OHD$_3$.

The conclusion from these observations is that both calcium supplements and oestrogens have a role to play in the management of post-menopausal osteoporosis, at least in those cases with normal calcium absorption, but the most effective therapy overall seems to be a combination of hormones with 1α-OHD$_3$. This is probably better than hormone or calcium therapy alone because many of these patients suffer from calcium malabsorption. Vitamin D and 1α-OHD$_3$ by themselves *and in the doses used* appear to do more harm than good, probably because of the sensitivity of bone to the resorbing action of these compounds, though it is conceivable that it may be possible to find a dose level sufficient to correct malabsorption of calcium without being so large as to increase bone resorption.

Other Forms of Osteoporosis

Corticosteroid-induced osteoporosis is generally associated with malabsorption of calcium which responds to large doses of vitamin D or small doses of a vitamin D metabolite. Such therapy also lowers the urinary hydroxyproline. In post-menopausal women on corticosteroid therapy, among whom osteoporosis is particularly common, the low plasma androgen and oestrogen levels secondary to adrenocortical suppression probably constitute an additional risk factor and may call for oestrogen or androgen treatment.

Osteoporosis is uncommon in men but it responds well to the combination of 1α-OHD$_3$ with hormones which has been so successful in post-menopausal osteoporosis, though the hormone used is, of course, testosterone rather than oestrogen. Our standard regime, therefore, is to give these patients $1-2$ μg daily of 1α-OHD$_3$ combined with weekly or fortnightly injections of $100-250$ mg of testosterone propionate. It must be emphasized, however, that this is empirical therapy because the pathogenesis of male osteoporosis is so poorly understood.

Osteomalacia

As already indicated, senile osteomalacia is associated with low plasma 25-OHD$_3$ levels and responds to vitamin D therapy. In the absence of gastrointestinal or renal disease, 1000 units of vitamin D daily is probably sufficient to cure this osteomalacia but it is our practice to give rather larger doses, of the order of $5000-10\,000$ units daily, because simple correction of vitamin D deficiency is not generally sufficient to correct malabsorption of calcium in older people. It seems likely that calcium supplements are also indicated to prevent the osteomalacia developing into osteoporosis.

CONCLUSIONS

Age-related bone loss in women starts at or about the time of the menopause, affects trabecular more than cortical bone and continues to the end of life. In men, the process starts later and proceeds more slowly. The dominant factor in post-menopausal loss of bone apears to be an increase in bone resorption, but in men there may be some decline in bone formation. Distal forearm fractures and vertebral compression fractures can be attributed to excessive loss of trabecular bone, and low trabecular bone mass is a striking feature of pertrochanteric femoral fractures but transcervical fractures are more likely to be due to cortical thinning. About 25 per cent of the female population suffer one or more of these fractures by age 80, and perhaps half this proportion of men. Malabsorption of calcium is present in most forms of osteoporosis and hormonal deficiency can be identified as an additional risk factor in females though seldom in males. Vitamin D deficiency makes an increasing contribution to bone pathology in patients over 65 years of age and histological evidence of osteomalacia is found in about 25 per cent of femoral neck fracture cases.

REFERENCES

Aaron J. E. (1976) In: Nordin B. E. C. (ed.), *Histology and Micro-anatomy of Bone in Calcium Phosphate and Magnesium Metabolism.* London, Churchill Livingstone, p. 298.

Aaron J. E., Gallagher J. C., Anderson J. et al. (1974a) *Lancet* 1, 229.

Aaron J. E., Gallagher J. C. and Nordin B. E. C. (1974b) *Lancet* 2, 84.

Arnold J. S. (1973) *Clin. Endocrinol. Metabol.* 2, 221.

Baker H. W. G., Burger H. G., de Kretzer D. M. et al. (1976) *Clin. Endocrinol. (Oxf.)* 5, 349.

Barnett E. and Nordin B. E. C. (1960) *Clin. Radiol.* 11, 166.

Chesnut C. H., Nelp W. B. and Cervellen T. K. (1976) *Calcif. Tissue Res.* Suppl. 370.

Exton-Smith A. N. (1971) *Br. J. Hosp. Med.* 5, 639.

Exton-Smith A. N., Millard P. H., Payne P. R. et al. (1969) *Lancet* 2, 1153.

Faccini J. N., Exton-Smith A. N. and Boyde A. (1976) *Lancet* 1, 1089.

Gallagher J. C., Aaron J., Horsman A. et al. (1973a) *Clin. Endocrinol. Metabol.* 2, 293.

Gallagher J. C., Bulusu L. and Nordin B. E. C. (1973b) In: Frame B., Parfitt A. M., and Duncan H. (ed.), *Clinical Aspects of Metabolic Bone Disease.* Amsterdam, Excerpta Medica, p. 266.

Gallagher J. C. and Nordin B. E. C. (1974) In: Curry A. S. and Hewitt J. V. (ed.), *Calcium Metabolism and the Menopause in Biochemistry of Women.* Cleveland, CRC, p. 145.

Gallagher J. C., Riggs L., Eisman J. et al. (1976) *Clin. Res.* 24, 360A.

Gallagher J. C., Young M. M. and Nordin B. E. C. (1972) *Clin. Endocrinol. (Oxf.)* 1, 57.

Garn S. M. (1970) *The Earlier Gain and Later Loss of Cortical Bone.* Springfield, Thomas.

Heaney R. P. (1965) *Am. J. Med.* 33, 188.

Hillyard C. J., Stevenson J. C. and MacIntyre I. (1978) *Lancet* 1, 961.

Hodkinson H. M. (1971) *Gerontol. Clin. (Basel)* 13, 153.

Horsman A. B. (1976) In: Nordin B. E. C. (ed.), *Calcium, Phosphate and Magnesium Metabolism.* Edinburgh, Churchill Livingstone, p. 357.

Horsman A., Gallagher J. C., Simpson M. et al. (1977a) *Br. Med. J.* 2, 789.

Horsman A., Simpson M., Kirby P. A. et al. (1977b) *Br. J. Radiol.* 50, 504.

Jasani C., Nordin B. E. C., Smith D. A. et al. (1965) *Proc. R. Soc. Med.* 58, 441.

Jenkins D. H. R., Roberts J. G., Webster D. et al. (1973) *J. Bone Joint Surg.* **55B**, 575.

Jowsey J., Riggs B. L., Kelly P. J. et al. (1972) *Am. J. Med.* **53**, 43.

Klotz H. P., Delorne M. L., Ochoa F. et al. (1975) *Sem. Hôp. Paris* **51**, 1333.

Knowelden J., Buhr A. J. and Dunbar O. (1964) *Br. J. Soc. Prev. Med.* **18**, 130.

Lindsay R., Aitken J. M., Anderson J. B. et al. (1976) *Lancet* **1**, 1038.

Marshall D. H., Crilly R. G. and Nordin B. E. C. (1977) *Br. Med. J.* **2**, 1177.

Marshall D. H. and Nordin B. E. C. Unpublished work.

Melsen F., Melsen B., Mosekilde L. et al. (1978) *Acta Pathol. Microbiol. Scand.* **86**, 70.

Meunier P., Courpron P., Edouard C. et al. (1973) *Clin. Endocrinol. Metabol.* **2**, 239.

Newton-John H. F. and Morgan D. B. (1970) *Clin. Orthop.* **71**, 229.

Nordin B. E. C. (1976) *Calcium, Phosphate and Magnesium Metabolism.* Edinburgh, Churchill Livingstone.

Nordin B. E. C., Horsman A., Brook R. et al. (1976) *Clin. Endocrinol. Metabol.* **5**, Suppl. 353s.

O'Driscoll M. (1973) *J. Bone Joint Surg.* **55B**, 882.

Recker R. R., Saville P. D. and Heaney R. O. (1977) *Ann. Intern. Med.* **87**, 649.

Riggs B. L., Jowsey J., Kelly P. J. et al. (1973) *Clin. Endocrinol. Metabol.* **2**, 317.

Saville P. D. (1965) *J. Bone Joint Surg.* **47A**, 492.

Sissons H. A., Holley K. J. and Heighway J. (1967) In: Hioco D. J. (ed.), *L'osteomalacie*. Paris, Masson.

Smith R. W. and Rizek J. (1966) *Clin. Orthop.* **45**, 31.

Smith R. W. and Walker R. R. (1964) *Science* **145**, 156.

Stamp T. C. B., and Round J. M. (1974) *Nature* **247**, 563.

Trotter M., Broman G. E. and Peterson R. R. (1960) *J. Bone Joint Surg.* **42A**, 50.

Weaver J. K. and Chalmers J. (1966) *J. Bone Joint Surg.* **48A**, 289.

12. THE EPIDEMIOLOGY OF DIABETES
H. Keen and J. H. Fuller

THE DIABETIC SYNDROME

A systematic influence of advancing age on carbohydrate metabolism, seen in rising plasma glucose concentration and in the progressively increasing plasma glucose response to oral carbohydrate loading, has been appreciated for many decades (Spence, 1921; Marshall, 1931). A key question is whether to equate this increasing glucose intolerance with the evolution of a treatable, definable, deleterious disease state, diabetes mellitus, or whether to regard it as an expected and benign consequence of ageing, therapeutic meddling with which may be misguided and even damaging to the individual; or whether both these interpretations apply. When the hyperglycaemia and glucose intolerance are accompanied by such symptoms as thirst, polyuria, pruritus vulvae or visual changes the operational question is readily answerable; the metabolic abnormality is very likely to be responsible for the symptoms and treatment will usually effectively relieve them. There is also in the elderly a continuing incidence of new cases of the severe, potentially lethal, ketoacidotic form of diabetes mellitus (often misnamed 'juvenile onset') for which prompt insulin treatment is lifesaving. Life-threatening diabetes may also present in the elderly with the state of non-ketotic, hyperglycaemic, hyperosmolality, sometimes in coma and frequently lethal, even when recognized and energetically treated (Alberti and Nattrass, 1978).

However, these latter clear-cut metabolic syndromes are the exception in the elderly; it is the large number of older people with asymptomatic or oligosymptomatic hyperglycaemia, often coming to light by chance as the result of routine screening biochemistry, in whom the diagnostic and therapeutic dilemma arises: whether to treat or not to treat? There is still no conclusive answer to this question, though information from a number of sources has accrued in recent years which begins to clarify the issue.

POPULATION STUDIES

The clear evidence of increasing average blood glucose concentrations in successively older samples of the general population, measured after overnight fasting and particularly after glucose loading either by the oral (O'Sullivan et al., 1971; Genuth et al., 1976) or the intravenous (Crockford et al., 1966; Cerasi and Luft, 1967) route, is well documented in the

146

literature (Andres and Tobin, 1974). Our own study of systematically performed oral glucose tolerance tests, carried out upon an age and sex stratified random sample of people, not known to be diabetic, cooperating in the town-wide Bedford Survey of 1962 (Sharp et al., 1964) is illustrated in *Fig.* 12.1 and represents the findings of others in many parts of the

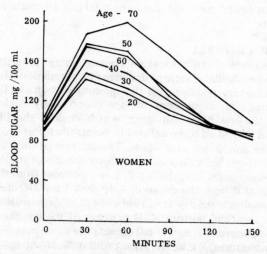

Fig. 12.1. Mean blood sugar values fasting (0) and at 30, 60, 90, 120 and 150 min after 50 g oral glucose load in a stratified random sample of the Bedford population cooperating in a screening survey for diabetes in 1962. Known diabetics and subjects with illnesses or taking medication known to affect glucose tolerance excluded. Capillary blood sugar measured by Auto-analyser ferricyanide reductiometric method. The progressive impairment of glucose tolerance with decades of age in this cross-sectional comparison is obvious. The mean curve of the 70–79 year decade in these ostensibly normal ambulant women itself met the British Diabetic Association definition for diabetes mellitus. Between 40 and 50 subjects in each decade.

world (though with two notable exceptions discussed later). Mean glucose tolerance curve values rise successively with decades of age and a steadily increasing proportion of the responses qualify for a diagnosis of diabetes as defined by the British Diabetic Association (Fitzgerald and Keen, 1964), or by many of the other national and professional bodies which have set diagnostic criteria (West, 1975).

There is no real evidence that the higher glucose values seen increasingly frequently with advancing age are other than the upper extreme of a positively skewed 'normal' (or better, log-normal) distribution of values. Nevertheless, the observation is also compatible with the hypothesis that a distinct subpopulation of diabetics is emerging with increasing age. These 'glycaemic outliers' may differ only quantitatively from the rest of the elderly population, or they may carry some qualitatively distinct diabeto-genic trait, 'released' by age. Lauvaux and Staquet (1970) argued the latter case on the evidence that the top fifth percentile boundary of the distribu-tion rose faster with age than the median or lower percentile boundaries. However, this observation may only indicate that higher values rise faster with age than lower ones and does not establish a qualitative difference between them.

DIAGNOSTIC CRITERIA

Few published sets of criteria make allowance for age in setting diagnostic limit levels. The calculated rates of diabetes in a population, therefore, vary (and may do so very widely) with the age composition and the diagnostic criteria selected. An adjustment for age proposed by Andres (1971) is based upon the use of a nomogram which enables the blood glucose position of an individual to be defined in percentile terms according to age and sex in the population as a whole. Though this permits one to define the position of an individual in relation to the concentration of blood glucose which separates, say, the top 5, 3 or 1 per cent from the rest of the population, it still begs the question – do they have diabetes mellitus or not? If one applies a strictly statistical definition of normality (i.e. mean ± 2 s.d), the top (and bottom) 2–3 per cent of the distribution will, by definition, be abnormal (i.e. will fall outside the mean plus or minus twice the standard deviation). However, great caution should be used in applying normal distribution criteria to populations of uncorrected blood glucose concentration which are notably positively skewed and become increasingly so as age advances.

The diagnostic problem is further complicated by the degree of variation in glucose tolerance when remeasured from time to time in the same person under apparently standardized conditions (McDonald et al., 1965), a variability of response which is not obviously related to age. Further problems arise from lack of standardization, such technical factors as the size of the carbohydrate load employed, the use of whole blood (capillary or venous) or plasma and the choice of chemical method for glucose assay. The degree and effects of the prevailing lack of agreement was documented by West (1975). The variation in criteria applied by diabetes experts, canvassed as to their own diagnostic practices, if applied to a single popu-lation of blood glucose responses would generate estimated diabetes prevalence rates varying between 2 and 73 per cent!

Recent discussions on revised blood glucose criteria for the diagnosis of diabetes (DM) and the introduction of a band of 'impaired glucose toler-ance' (IGT) short of DM may help to resolve the present confusions about hyperglycaemia in the elderly (Keen et al., 1979a). Most countries support proposals that blood glucose values diagnosing DM from the oral glucose tolerance test should be set higher than before. This would considerably reduce the numbers of those diagnosed as diabetic from the glucose tolerance test (GTT), particularly among the elderly. However, the range of glucose intolerance thereby freed from the diabetic category (e.g. two hour post glucose load values of 7–11 mmol/l), the IGT band, is not meant to be neglected (IGT – *see Table* 12.1). This borderline degree of glucose intolerance indicates increased susceptibility to atherosclerotic disease and a greater risk of metabolic deterioration to diabetes.

Table 12.1. Suggested criteria for the diagnosis of diabetes mellitus (DM) and impaired glucose tolerance (IGT) from the oral glucose tolerance test

---

Proposed Guidelines for Diagnosis (stated in terms of venous whole blood, true glucose measurements, following a 75 g oral glucose load where appropriate):

    1. Diabetes mellitus is diagnosed when
        (a) The fasting blood glucose concentration equals or exceeds 7 mmol/l (126 mg/dl) on more than one occasion.
        (b)* The blood glucose concentration two hours after a 75 g oral glucose load equals or exceeds 10 mmol/l (180 mg/dl) irrespective of the fasting concentration.

*N.B. This differs from the NIH Diabetes Data Group proposal which at present also requires a value of 10 mmol/l or more preceding the two-hour value for clinical diagnosis though not necessarily for epidemiological purposes.

    2. Impaired glucose tolerance (IGT) exists when the two hour blood glucose concentration falls between 7 and 10 mmol/l. Action with IGT depends upon individual circumstances except during pregnancy when it has the same immediate significance as a diagnosis of diabetes.

POPULATION DIFFERENCES

In two unusual populations, the Pima Indians described by Bennett and his colleagues (Hamman et al., 1978) and the Micronesian population of the island of Nauru (Zimmet and Taft, 1978) the prevalence of diabetes in people achieving and surpassing age 50 is about 50 per cent. The population distribution of two hour post load plasma glucose values progressively separates out into a bimodal form with increasing age. In this population diabetes has been defined as the intersection of the two subdistributions. Bennett has argued that the skewed distributions of Westernized populations are *formes frustes* of this Pima bimodality.

Observations and arguments on the effects of increasing age derived from obese, inbred populations of Amerindians or Pacific Islanders cannot unreservedly be applied to the much more outbred, leaner populations of the West; and there are no metabolic studies of Western populations as faithfully observed as the Pima.

BORDERLINE DIABETES AND ITS EVOLUTION

Observations that we have made over a ten-year period of a group of individuals selected because of their 'borderline' impairments of glucose

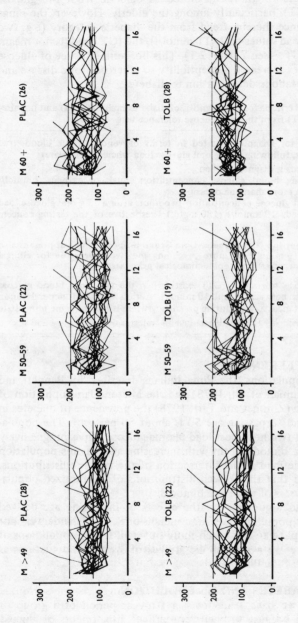

Fig. 12.2. Course over 10 years (examinations 0–17, see abscissae) of blood glucose measured 2 h after 50 g oral glucose load (taken in the afternoon after a day-long fast). Males from a population of so-called 'borderline diabetics' (b.d.) (i.e. found at survey to have whole blood capillary blood sugar values > 120 mg/dl < 200 mg/dl) detected in Bedford Diabetes Detection Survey of 1962. Double-blind random allocation to treatment with tolbutamide 0·5 g b.d. or indistinguishable placebo.

tolerance show many patterns of metabolic change with time. Some have shown slow, smooth deterioration of tolerance; in others there has been abrupt development of symptomatic, even insulin-requiring, diabetes; in many others glucose intolerance has remitted, apparently spontaneously, to a state of unequivocal normality (Jarrett et al., 1979) (*Fig.* 12.2).

Some indication of the varied patterns of blood sugar behaviour over ten years for men can be seen in *Fig.* 12.2 which shows a time trend 'spaghettogram' of blood sugar in three age cohorts (under 50, 50—59 and 60 and over). Half of the group was treated with tolbutamide, 0·5 g twice a day, the other half receiving a placebo tablet on a 'double-blind' basis. There is no greater trend for older than younger subjects to 'worsen to diabetes' (i.e. to exceed the upper limit of the borderline category, 200 mg/dl 2h after 50 g oral glucose). The oldest of the three groups appears to maintain a more stable position within the IGT category compared with the youngest group, a high proportion of which, with or without tolbutamide, regresses to normoglycaemia.

GLYCAEMIA AND AGE, INSULIN RESPONSES

Our own studies in normal population samples (Boyns et al., 1969) suggested that, though post-glucose load glycaemia clearly increases with age, insulinaemic responses show relatively little change (*Table* 12.2). In a

Table 12.2. Beecham study: Mean plasma insulin (microunits/ml) by age and sex

Age (yrs)	Number M/F	Fasting insulin		2 hr insulin (after 50 g oral glucose)	
		M	F	M	F
24	24/22	15·2	19·0	17·9	33·3
25—34	22/22	14·7	17·6	16·7	31·2
35—44	20/22	15·7	14·9	20·8	24·8
45—54	22/23	16·6	14·6	24·6	23·7
55+	21/24	12·5	16·5	22·2	29·2

From Boyns et al. (1969).

group of older people selected because of strictly normal glucose tolerance (Chlouverakis et al., 1967) the corresponding insulin response values were higher than in a comparably aged group with IGT (borderline diabetes), suggesting that normal tolerance is retained in the elderly only in the presence of, perhaps at the expense of, higher circulating insulin concentrations. Whether this altered relationship points to an increasing peripheral resistance to the effects of insulin with age, or to lessened sensitivity of the ageing pancreatic B cell to the glycaemic stimulus, has been widely argued.

Most recently a change in the partitioning of insulin between plasma and extravascular sites has been described by McGuire et al. (1979).

FACTORS INFLUENCING GLUCOSE TOLERANCE
Many factors are known to impair glucose tolerance and these may assume relatively greater importance in older people. They include physical inactivity, degree of adiposity, the presence of other physical disorders and the taking of certain medications (Siperstein, 1975). Each of these is likely to have a greater influence on the diminishingly adaptive homeostatic mechanisms of the elderly and should be considered in any population-based appraisal. The widespread use of thiazide diuretics in the treatment of dependent oedema, hypertension and congestive heart failure, for example, contribute to an unknown extent to the sum of glucose intolerance. The trend to increasing adiposity with age is well established (Montegriffo, 1971). Even though total body weight may not increase, the proportion of fat grows at the expense of the lean body mass (Moore et al., 1963). However, adiposity *per se* is probably of limited diabetogenic potential. The fat person is much more likely to be diabetic if related to a late-onset diabetic, particularly a thin one (Baird, 1972). The underlying genetic factors which confer susceptibility to non-insulin dependent diabetes in the presence of adiposity (Keen et al., 1979b) are poorly understood.

Cases of acute-onset, insulin dependent diabetes starting in the elderly differ aetiologically and genetically from the much commoner oligo-symptomatic, non insulin dependent variety with an excess of the HLA antigens characterizing insulin dependent diabetes of juvenile onset. Few youthful-onset cases of diabetes survive to present problems in their geriatric years. Long-term survivors, for reasons at present unknown, are peculiarly spared the worst of the vascular and tissue complications of the disease (Oakley et al., 1974). Some of them may be the so-called MODY (maturity onset diabetes of youth) variety (Tattersall and Fajans, 1975) the larger proportion of whom, as well as showing a clearly dominant genetic pattern of transmission of diabetes, also enjoy comparative freedom from diabetic complications. An interesting recent twist to this story has been taken by the identification of the liability to flush with alcohol after chlorpropamide (CPAF — chlorpropamide alcohol flush) as a probable marker for a particular subclass of non-insulin dependent diabetics (NIDDs), found across the whole age range. This flushing subgroup of NIDDs has a strong first degree family history of diabetes and also appears less susceptible to the more advanced forms of diabetic retinopathy (Leslie et al., 1979). It has also been claimed (Irvine et al., 1977a) that a subset of apparently typical, older-onset NIDDs, characterized by the presence of circulating islet-cell antibodies, are more likely to show metabolic deterioration with time and to come to require insulin treatment. They also resemble typical insulin dependent diabetics (IDDs) in their HLA constitution.

The often quoted possibility of late onset diabetes mellitus arising from pancreatic ischaemia due to vascular disease is difficult to evaluate as little satisfactory data are available.

CASE PRESENTATION
Another approach to diabetes epidemiology in the elderly is to observe the patterns of prevalence of known diabetics and also to consider the access of newly diagnosed cases. It is likely to be some second factor, often some other disease, which brings a hitherto unsuspected diabetic state to attention. This phenomenon of linked diagnosis is responsible for much of the apparent clinical association between diabetes and other disorders.

The US house-to-house survey of known diabetics (US National Health Survey, 1964) showed a rapid rise in prevalence after age 60 which corresponds with the peak of presentation at around 60 years approximately at the Birmingham Diabetic Clinic (Malins, 1968). The timing of this late age-peak, independent of the age/sex structure of the population, varies somewhat in different groups; but it is not clear whether this represents a true variation in the age of onset of metabolic disorder or in patterns of health care in different social groupings.

MORBID ASSOCIATIONS OF HYPERGLYCAEMIA
The clinical significance of hyperglycaemia or glucose intolerance in the elderly is to be assessed from observations of its clinical consequences. These may be immediate, such as the presence of symptoms attributable to hyperglycaemia like thirst and polyuria, weight loss, pruritus vulvae, etc.; or they may be longer-term, as for example with the evolution of morbidity and mortality from arterial disease, the retinal and renal consequences of microvascular disease, or the development of neuropathy and cataract. Mortality rates for the newly found diabetics, borderline diabetics and matched normoglycaemic controls from the 10-year follow-up of the Bedford study are shown in *Table* 12.3 for deaths certified to coronary heart disease (CHD), all cardiovascular disease (CVD), and all causes. For both the 40–59 years and 60+ years age groups, mortality rates for CHD and CVD are substantially higher in the diabetic than in the control groups in both sexes, though, in these comparatively small numbers, achieving significance only in the women. The borderline diabetic groups generally have intermediate rates. The ratio of mortality in older compared with younger groups suggests that diabetes reduces the influence of ageing by increasing rates in the younger subjects (Keen et al., 1965).

MORTALITY AND AGE IN DIABETICS
Trends in mortality rates for diabetes as underlying cause have been discussed by Reid and Evans (1970) for England and Wales for the period

Table 12.3. Bedford study: 10-year mortality rates by age

	Normoglycaemic controls		Borderline diabetics		Newly found diabetics	
	M	F	M	F	M	F
Numbers: 40–59yr	50	31	58	42	17	31
60+ yr	41	42	47	61	29	35
1. Coronary Heart Disease						
(a) 40–59yr	4·0*(2)†	0(0)	5·2(3)	4·8(2)	17·6(3)	9·7(3)
(b) 60+ yr	12·2(5)	2·4(1)	23·4(11)	16·4(10)	17·2(5)	22·9(8)
Mortality ratio (b/a)	3·1	–	4·4	3·4	1·0	2·4
2. Cardiovascular Disease						
(a) 40–59 yr	8·0(4)	0(0)	6·9(4)	9·5(4)	17·6(3)	12·9(4)
(b) 60+ yr	22·0(9)	11·9(5)	36·2(17)	31·1(19)	41·4(12)	40·0(14)
Mortality ratio (b/a)	2·8	–	5·2	3·3	2·4	3·1
3. All Causes						
(a) 40–59 yr	10·0(5)	3·2(1)	8·6(5)	16·7(7)	29·4(5)	12·9(4)
(b) 60+ yr	36·6(15)	16·7(7)	48·9(23)	42·6(26)	48·3(14)	51·4(18)
Mortality ratio (b/a)	3·7	5·2	5·7	2·6	1·6	4·0

* 10-year mortality rate per 100.
† Number of deaths.
From unpublished data (in preparation).

from 1901 to 1966. In the period from 1955 to 1966, death rates over the age of 35 remained relatively stable for women, but showed a steady rise among men. More recent data for the period 1968–1976 [Office of Population Censuses and Surveys (OPCS), 1978] suggest that for women above 60 years there has actually been a progressive fall in diabetes mortality. Rates for men have levelled off above the age of 65, but have continued to rise for the age range 45–64 years. Diabetes may be mentioned on the death certificate but is not always coded as the 'underlying cause of death' and its contribution to mortality is then difficult to evaluate. In the period 1920–30, 91 per cent of all certificates mentioning diabetes coded it as the 'underlying cause'. In 1976 the proportion had fallen to 23 per cent, being so ascribed mainly in those dying under age 50 (Fuller and Goldblatt, 1979). Most of the deaths in diabetics late in life are likely to be cardiovascular in cause and there is nothing distinctive about arterial disease of heart, leg or brain in the diabetic. Nevertheless, the influence of diabetes is clearly apparent from the fact that amputation for gangrene is many times likelier to occur in a diabetic than a non-diabetic (Crofford, 1976).

MULTIPLE CAUSE CODING ANALYSIS

The contribution of diabetes to mortality can be better assessed by the method of multiple cause coding of death certificates now being undertaken in UK by the OPCS (Fuller and Goldblatt, 1979). Using this method a 'proportional registration ratio' (PRR) has been calculated (observed/expected deaths X 100) for various underlying causes of death for the year 1976 in England and Wales. The analysis in *Table* 12.4 excludes those

Table 12.4. Conditional proportional registration ratios (England and Wales, 1976) for mentions of diabetes by selected underlying cause

Underlying Cause	Males		Females	
	45–64 yr	65+ yrs	45–64 yr	65+ yrs
1. Malignant neoplasms of digestive organs (150–159)*	44	58	37	45
2. Malignant neoplasms of trachea, bronchus and lung (162)*	39	41	14	35
3. Ischaemic heart disease (410–414)*	131	122	229	129
4. Other heart disease (420–429)*	183	109	168	101
5. Cerebrovascular disease (430–438)*	206	152	169	126
6. Pneumonia (480–486)*	150	130	202	112
7. Bronchitis and emphysema (490–492)*	42	57	35	62
8. Nephritis and nephrosis (580–584)*	150	163	232	138

*ICD Codes.
From Fuller J. H. and Goldblatt P. (1979).

certificates where diabetes was coded as underlying cause and therefore describes 'conditional PRRs'. The conditional PRRs are low (i.e. rates in deaths with diabetes mention lower than overall rates) for certain neoplasms and bronchitis and emphysema. For the vascular disease groupings of underlying cause, ischaemic heart disease, other heart disease and cerebrovascular disease, the PRRs are generally increased, but far less in the older age range (65+ years) than the younger (45–64 years); and the same is true for pneumonia as underlying cause.

PROSPECTIVE STUDIES

In their prospective study of diabetic mortality in Edinburgh, Shenfield et al. (1979) examined the death rates in over three thousand diabetics of all ages identified as living in Edinburgh and district on 1 January, 1968.

Analysis of the 1272 (41 per cent) patients who died over the subsequent eight years confirmed the increased vulnerability of diabetic women whose rates equalled those for men. The excess risk of death in the elderly diabetic was independent of the increased risk due to diabetes duration and was unrelated to the form of treatment received. The independent contribution of age (A), diabetes duration (D) and form of treatment (T) to the probability of dying (P) over the eight years of study could be expressed by the following equation:

$$\text{Log } P/(1 - P) = 1 \cdot 97 - A - D - T.$$

Age	(A)	Duration	(D)	Treatment	(T)
10–39	4·95	0–4	0·39	Insulin	0·39
40–49	3·35	5–9	0·36	Oral agents	0·00
50–59	2·51	10–14	0·22	Diet only	0·00
60–69	1·64	15+	0·00		
70–79	1·11				
80+	0·00				

In simple comparisons of mortality rates by sex and age group between their diabetic cohort and the general population of Scotland, the overall risk in men of 60–69 was 1·65; 70–79, 1·35; and 80+, 1·01: and in women 3·03, 1·98 and 1·16 respectively.

In several other studies comparing the mortality experience of diabetic clinic populations with that of the general population (Hayward and Lucena, 1965; Kessler, 1971) the ratio of death rates in diabetics to rates in the general population falls progressively with increasing age groups, especially in those aged 65 or more, but always remains greater than unity up to the age of 80. In studies based upon insurance statistics (Bale and Entmacher, 1977), the life expectancy of diabetics only approaches that of the general population at age 80 or more for men and 75 or more for women. In the study of Goodkin (1975), the life expectancy of diabetics applying for life insurance was 17 years less than that of the standard US insured population when the age at diabetes diagnosis was 15 years or less, but only 5 years shorter for age at diagnosis of 60–70 years.

Thus all these studies indicate that, although mortality rates remain increased in Western diabetics above the age of 65, selectively for cardiovascular causes, excess mortality is considerably less in those diagnosed late in life than in those diagnosed earlier.

MICROVASCULAR DISEASE

There is comparatively little reliable evidence of the impact of microvascular disease, the specific angiopathy of diabetes, on the elderly diabetic. *Table* 12.5 shows the prevalence of evidence of microangiopathy (retinopathy and proteinuria) and of cardiac ischaemia and peripheral arterial disease in newly diagnosed diabetics attending King's College Hospital,

Table 12.5. Prevalence of vascular disease in newly diagnosed Caucasian diabetics (King's College Hospital, London, May 1974 to April 1979)

		Age group			
		25–54 yr	55–64 yr	65–74 yr	75+ yr
1. Background retinopathy	M	9(5·9%)	18(12·4%)	5(5·5%)	3(8·8%)
	F	3(4·1%)	11(10·1%)	8(6·1%)	4(5·0%)
2. Proliferative retinopathy	M	3(2·0%)	0(–)	0(–)	0(–)
	F	0(–)	1(0·9%)	1(0·8%)	0(–)
3. Proteinuria	M	8(5·2%)	11(7·6%)	7(7·7%)	2(5·9%)
	F	3(4·1%)	5(4·6%)	8(6·1%)	6(7·5%)
4. Cataract	M	3(2·0%)	8(5·5%)	9(9·9%)	5(14·7%)
	F	0(–)	2(1·8%)	21(16·0%)	35(43·8%)
5. Past history of myocardial infarction	M	4(2·6%)	8(5·5%)	7(7·7%)	0(–)
	F	0(–)	4(3·7%)	3(2·3%)	2(2·5%)
6. Angina pectoris	M	4(2·6%)	9(6·2%)	9(9·9%)	2(5·9%)
	F	1(1·4%)	6(5·5%)	6(4·6%)	7(8·8%)
7. Intermittent claudication	M	4(2·6%)	9(6·2%)	8(8·8%)	2(5·9%)
	F	0(–)	3(2·8%)	4(3·1%)	1(1·2%)

From Soler et al. (1969).

London for the first time in the period May 1974 to April 1979. In both sexes, the prevalence of background retinopathy at diagnosis is higher in the 55–64 years age group than in the younger age group (25–54 years) but thereafter is somewhat lower in the later age groups. Soler et al. (1969) found no rise in the frequency of retinopathy with age at diagnosis when diabetes was found after age 50.

Positivity rates for clinical proteinuria (Bromphenol blue strip test) show a small upward trend with age at diagnosis in women but not in men. The findings of diabetic microangiopathy at the time of diagnosis in the elderly strongly suggests the existence of many years of unsuspected diabetes before its clinical discovery (Soler et al., 1969). The pressure for population screening for diabetes was based upon the (as yet unsubstantiated) view that early discovery and correction of the metabolic fault would delay or prevent the evolution of the microvascular complications and associated disability. It is the lack of evidence supporting this view that has reduced enthusiasm for this approach to pre-emptive diagnosis. The plateau in retinopathy prevalence at diagnosis after the age of 50 years suggests either a fairly constant prior period of unrecognized metabolic disturbance, regardless of age, or that hyperglycaemia is less damaging to retinovascular structures in the elderly than in the middle-aged. Caird's observations on retinopathy in known diabetics (Caird et al., 1969) do not bear out this latter interpretation, for he found that the increase in prevalence with duration was greater, and the rate of worsening more rapid, in older than in younger diabetics. The pathogenesis of the diabetes and therefore its consequences might differ in these different age groups. Adiposity, for instance, becomes a less dominating presenting feature as age of diabetes detection rises (Keen, 1975). The intensity of the metabolic abnormality in respect of area of glycaemic excess during the day or the degree of hyperinsulinaemia (as suggested by Turkington and Weindling, 1978) may also modify susceptibility to microangiopathy.

In numerical terms by far the largest proportion of those newly registering blind from diabetic retinopathy in the UK comes from those aged 60 or more. For some of these this is the culmination of many years of known prior diabetes; but a considerable proportion will have been of short known duration and may even have presented with visual symptoms due to retinopathy. Visual loss due to diabetic retinopathy in the elderly is usually of the non-proliferative, maculopathic variety (*Interim Report of a Multicentre Controlled Study*, 1975), but this type is susceptible to treatment with photocoagulation and perhaps to treatment with prophylactic hypolipidaemic agents (Kohner and Dollery, 1975).

THE MECHANISM OF DIABETIC COMPLICATIONS

Much of the tissue pathology of diabetes has been likened to premature ageing processes. Cataract occurs at an earlier age in diabetics (Beckett and Hobbs, 1961) and *Table* 12.5 shows the prevalence of cataract with age at diagnosis in the King's diabetics. Autoimmune phenomena associated with ageing in the general population occur earlier in the insulin dependent diabetic (Irvine et al., 1977b) though not in the non-insulin dependent variety. Premature development of arterial disease (Jarrett and Keen, 1975) and accelerated thickening of capillary basement membrane (Kilo et al., 1972) are consistent with this general hypothesis, as is the accelerated ageing of collagen in the diabetic (Hamlin and Kohn, 1972). The replicative programme, and so survival *in vitro*, of fibroblasts derived from diabetic subjects is diminished (Goldstein et al., 1969). The accelerated demise of cells of the microvascular wall has been proposed as an explanation for the laminated thickening of capillary basement membrane (Vracko and Benditt, 1974). The impaired glucose homeostasis and glucose intolerance of the elderly diabetic may itself be a result of relatively early development of ageing process of the islet B-cell, with loss of sensitivity to the glycaemic stimulus or of total insulin secretory capacity of the B-cell mass.

ACKNOWLEDGEMENTS

The authors wish to express their appreciation to the following for their help in the preparation of this chapter: Dr Gilliam Watkins, King's College Hospital Diabetic Clinic; Mr Peter McCartney and Mrs Briony Thomas, Unit for Metabolic Medicine, Guy's Hospital; and Mr Peter Goldblatt, Medical Statistics Division, Office of Population Censuses and Surveys.

REFERENCES

Alberti K. G. M. M. and Nattrass M. (1978) *Med. Clin. North Am.* **62**, 799.

Andres R. (1971) *Med. Clin. North Am.* **55**, 835.

Andres R. and Tobin J. D. (1974) *Adv. Exp. Med. Biol.* **61**, 239.

Baird J. D. (1972) *Acta Diabetol. Lat.* **9**, Suppl. 1, 621.

Bale G. S. and Entmacher P. S. (1977) *Diabetes* **26**, 434.

Beckett A. G. and Hobbs H. E. (1961) *Br. Med. J.* **2**, 1605.

Boyns D. R., Crossley J. N., Abrams M. E. et al. (1969) *Br. Med. J.* **1**, 595.

Caird F. I., Pirie A. and Ramsell T. G. (1969) *Diabetes and the Eye.* Oxford and Edinburgh, Blackwell.

Cerasi E. and Luft R. (1967) *Acta Endocrinol.* **55**, 278.

Chlouverakis C., Jarrett R. J. and Keen H. (1967) *Lancet* **1**, 806.

Crockford P. M., Harbeck R. J. and Williams R. H. (1966) *Lancet* **1**, 465.

Crofford O. B. (1976) *Report of the National Commission on Diabetes*, vol. 1: *The Long-range Plan to Combat Diabetes*, No. (NIH) 76-1018. US Department of Health, Education and Welfare, Public Health Service, National Institutes of Health.

Fitzgerald M. G. and Keen H. (1964) *Br. Med. J.* **1**, 1568.

Fuller J. H. and Goldblatt P. (1979) In preparation.

Genuth S. M., Houser H. B., Carter J. R. et al. (1976) *Diabetes* **25**, 1110.

Goldstein S., Littlefield J. W. and Soeldner J. S. (1969) *Proc. Natl Acad. Sci. USA* **64**, 155.

Goodkin G. (1975) *J. Occup. Med.* **17**, 716.

Hamlin C. R. and Kohn N. R. (1972) *Exp. Gerontol.* **7**, 377.

Hamman R. F., Bennett P. H. and Miller M. (1978) *Adv. Metab. Disord.* **9**, 49.

Hayward R. E. and Lucena B. C. (1965) *J. Inst. Actuaries* **91**, 286.

Interim Report of a Multicentre Controlled Study (1975) *Lancet* **2**, 1110.

Irvine W. J., McCallum C. J., Gray R. S. et al. (1977a) *Lancet* **1**, 1025.

Irvine W. J., McCallum C. J., Gray R. S. et al. (1977b) *Diabetes* **26**, 138.

Jarrett R. J. and Keen H. (1975) In: Keen H. and Jarrett R. J. (ed.), *Complications of Diabetes.* London, Edward Arnold, p. 179.

Jarrett R. J., Keen H., Fuller J. H. et al. (1979) *Diabetologia* **16**, 25.

Keen H. (1975) *Recent Advances in Obesity Research.* Vol. 1, London, Newman, p. 116.

Keen H., Jarrett R. J. and Alberti K. G. M. M. (1979a) *Diabetologia* **16**, 283.

Keen H., Jarrett R. J., Thomas B. J. et al. (1979) In: Vague J. and Vague P. H. (ed.), *Diabetes and Obesity.* Excerpta Medica International Congress Series 454. Amsterdam and Oxford. p. 91.

Keen H., Rose G., Pyke D. A. et al. (1965) *Lancet* **2**, 505.

Kessler I. I. (1971) *Am. J. Med.* **51**, 715.

Kilo C., Vogler N. and Williamson J. R. (1972) *Diabetes* **21**, 881.

Kohner E. M. and Dollery C. T. (1975) In: Keen H. and Jarrett R. J. (ed.), *Complications of Diabetes.* London, Edward Arnold, p. 7.

Lauvaux J. P. and Staquet M. (1970) *Diabetologia* **6**, 414.

Leslie R. D. G., Barnett A. H. and Pyke D. A. (1979) *Lancet* **1**, 997.

McDonald G. W., Fisher G. F. and Burnham C. (1965) *Diabetes* **14**, 473.

McGuire E. A., Tobin J. D., Berman M. et al. (1979) *Diabetes* **28**, 110.

Malins J. (1968) *Clinical Diabetes Mellitus.* London, Eyre & Spottiswoode, p. 52.

Marshall F. W. (1931) *Q. J. Med.* **24**, 257.

Montegriffo V. M. E. (1971) *Postgrad. Med. J.* June Suppl., 418.

Moore F. D., Olesen K. H., McMurrey J. D. et al. (1963) *The Body Cell Mass and its Supporting Environment.* Philadelphia, Saunders, p. 163.

Oakley W. G., Pyke D. A., Tattersall R. B. et al. (1974) *Q. J. Med.* **43**, 145.

Office of Population Censuses and Surveys (1978) *Mortality Surveillance, 1968–76, England and Wales,* London, HMSO.

O'Sullivan J. B., Mahan C. M., Freelender A. E. et al. (1971) *J. Clin. Endocrinol. Metab.* **33**, 619.
Reid D. D. and Evans J. G. (1970) *Br. Med. Bull.* **26**, 191.
Sharp C. L., Butterfield W. J. H. and Keen H. (1964) *Proc. R. Soc. Med.* **57**, 193.
Shenfield G. M., Elton R. A., Bhalla I. P. et al. (1979) *Diabete et Metabolisme* **5**, 149.
Siperstein M. D. (1975) *Adv. Intern. Med.* **20**, 297.
Soler N. G., Fitzgerald M. G., Malins J. M. et al. (1969) *Br. Med. J.* **3**, 567.
Spence J. C. (1921) *Q. J. Med.* **14**, 314.
Tattersall R. B. and Fajans S. S. (1975) *Diabetes* **24**, 44.
Turkington R. W. and Weindling H. K. (1978) *J. Am. Med. Assoc.* **240**, 833.
US National Health Survey (1964) No. 1000, Series 11, No. 2.
Vracko R. and Benditt E. D. (1974) *Am. J. Pathol.* **75**, 204.
West K. M. (1975) *Diabetes* **24**, 641.
Zimmet P. and Taft P. (1978) *Adv. Metab. Disord.* **9**, 225.

13. MANAGEMENT OF DIABETES AND ITS COMPLICATIONS
F. I. Caird

The basic objectives of the management of diabetes in old age are identical to those in youth and middle age, and comprise the control of symptoms and of the metabolic disorder itself in an attempt to prevent long-term complications. The evidence that these complications are related to diabetic control is reviewed below (p. 168), and if accepted must lead to the view that diabetes is significant whatever the age of the patient, and must never be neglected or ignored. Nevertheless the practical management of the individual patient must at all times take into account the realities of the situation, and in particular potentially relevant factors such as mental state, the degree of obesity, and the presence of complications and of other conditions which may affect the practicalities of treatment. Significant mental impairment in particular may make it almost impossible to carry out any plan of treatment. A compromise based on the practicable rather than the theoretically desirable may be a necessity.

NEWLY DISCOVERED DIABETES
The management of newly discovered diabetes in old age is based as at any age on diet, oral hypoglycaemic agents and insulin. Its most important single aspect is the education of the patient and those caring for him in the nature of the condition and the objectives of treatment.

Dietary Treatment
Dietary treatment should be advised for every old person in whom a definite diagnosis of diabetes is made. The common problems are the need for carbohydrate restriction and for weight reduction. Dietary surveys in the UK show that the energy intakes of most old people are more than adequate to maintain body weight, and that carbohydrate intakes average around 200 g per day (DHSS 1972; MacLeod et al., 1974). Reduction in carbohydrate intake to 120–150 g/d (or 100 g/d if the patient is obese), with maintenance of a normal protein and fat intake, and attention to other nutrients whose intake may be less than optimal (in particular ascorbic acid), is usually all that is necessary.

Dietary advice should be simple and flexible, should allow an adequate variety for the individual's own preferences and choices, and should avoid setting inappropriate dietary patterns (MacLeod and Caird, 1975). The principles should be explained not only to the patient, but also to relatives caring for him or living in the same house, and if necessary to those in charge of diets in institutions for the elderly. For the individual, advice is best given by a dietitian at a diabetic clinic, but could later well be reinforced at a health centre; health visitors can have an important rôle in this connection (MacLeod, 1970).

Unfortunately it is clear that the effectiveness of dietary advice as at present given is limited. Some 30 per cent of diabetics do not keep to their diets at all, a further 30 per cent make some gesture in the right direction, and only in the remainder does what is consumed bear a reasonable relation to what has been advised (Tunbridge and Wetherill, 1970). These difficulties may result in part from the higher cost of diabetic diets, and so the compliance of elderly patients might be expected to be less perfect than that of younger patients; this is apparently not so (Tunbridge and Wetherill, 1970). Another reason may be the great variation in the ways in which dietary advice is presented at clinics (Thomas et al., 1974). The commonest form of presentation is a single basic menu with spaces for amounts of carbohydrate-containing foods. Simplified diet sheets specifically for the elderly with large print and a minimum of detail are rarely provided. A suitable booklet offering a range of menus for elderly patients is that issued by the British Diabetic Association (1973).

Oral Hypoglycaemic Therapy

Oral hypoglycaemic therapy is indicated in a newly discovered elderly diabetic if dietary management does not result in reduction of hyperglycaemia and abolition of glycosuria within a few weeks, provided ketosis has never been present. It is usual to begin with a sulphonylurea, though in the obese a biguanide may be preferred, to encourage weight loss by its anorectic effect (Patel and Stowers, 1964). Some physicians begin treatment with a sulphonylurea before commencing dietary treatment, arguing that the more rapid control of symptoms makes subsequent compliance with dietary advice more likely. The problems presented by the findings of the University Diabetes Group Program (1970) are discussed below.

1. Sulphonylureas

Only three sulphonylureas will be discussed (tolbutamide, chlorpropamide, and glibenclamide). The other members of the group, such as acetohexamide, metahexamide, and glypizide, have no particular advantages. The lesser efficacy of tolbutamide and the need to give more than one dose per day in the majority of cases make it less satisfactory than chlorpropamide in the elderly, despite the greater risk of hypoglycaemia from impaired excretion of the latter.

Chlorpropamide should be begun in a single dose of 100 mg per day, and increased weekly by 100 mg increments if glycosuria persists, until a maximum of 500 mg/d is reached. The minimum number of tablets can then be achieved by the use of 250 mg tablets. A small number of patients develop hypoglycaemia on 100 mg of chlorpropamide per day; most of these can in fact be controlled by diet alone, but if drug therapy is truly necessary, tolbutamide 500 mg/d is preferable.

The principal problem with chlorpropamide therapy in the elderly is hypoglycaemia. Schen and Benaroya (1976) report 22 patients, of mean age 72 years, with five deaths. Factors predisposing to reduced food intake were definitely present in three cases, and perhaps five more, while renal function was impaired in four. In eight the dose of chlorpropamide was 500 mg/d or more. Careful selection of patients, limitation of dosage and prompt discontinuance of the drug if food intake falls are important aspects of treatment with chlorpropamide in old age.

A second mechanism of impairment of consciousness due to chlorpropamide is water intoxication (Garcia et al., 1971). There is doubt whether this is due to increased secretion of antidiuretic hormone, or to increased sensitivity of the renal tubules to normal amounts of circulating ADH (de Troyer and Demanet, 1976). Clinical improvement and disappearance of hyponatraemia are rapid once chlorpropamide is withdrawn.

If tolbutamide is preferred as oral therapy, it should be begun in a dose of 500 mg daily, and increased to three times daily; doses of more than 1·5 g/d are rarely effective. Glibenclamide is begun in a dose of 2·5 mg/d and the maximum useful dose is 20 mg/d.

A high proportion of elderly patients considered suitable for sulphonylurea treatment are satisfactorily controlled (Balodimos et al., 1966; Malins 1968). Failure within a few months is usually due to improper selection, dietary excess, inadequate dosage, or side effects such as a drug rash; while later, 'secondary' failure, occurring after many months or years, is relatively rare, especially with chlorpropamide (Cervantes-Amezcua et al., 1965). There is little benefit in substituting another sulphonylurea if drug failure occurs. The addition of a biguanide is much more likely to be successful.

2. *Biguanides*

Of the two biguanide drugs in common use, phenformin and metformin, there is no doubt that the latter is much to be preferred in the elderly. Phenformin produces considerably higher blood lactate concentrations both after glucose loads (Alexander and Marples, 1977) and exercise (Björntorp et al., 1978), and is thus more likely than metformin to result in lactic acidosis — a condition with a high mortality (Gale and Tattersall, 1976; Wise et al., 1976; Bergman et al., 1978). Lactic acidosis can develop very rapidly, and is particularly associated with renal impairment, high blood pressure, and cardiac failure — all common conditions in elderly diabetics (Gale and Tattersall 1976; Wise et al., 1976). Metformin should be given in doses of 500 mg once to three times per day. It may produce nausea, vomiting and occasionally diarrhoea at the beginning of treatment, and later weakness and malaise. About 10 per cent of patients need to discontinue treatment because of side effects (Malins, 1968).

A considerable proportion of elderly patients in whom sulphonylureas alone fail can be maintained on oral therapy by the addition of a biguanide (Bloom and Richards, 1961); but if the combination fails, there should be no hesitation in advising a change in insulin. Indeed Malins (1968) suggests that 'senile or demented patients who cannot be trusted to take tablets regularly' should, if at all possible, be treated from the outset with insulin, given by a member of the family or a nurse.

Insulin

Insulin is often necessary in elderly patients with acutely disordered diabetes, but is relatively rarely needed for purposes of long-term treatment. It is however advisable in patients in whom oral therapy fails, and there is a small group of thin elderly men whose diabetes is insulin-dependent from the first; it should never be thought that such diabetes does not occur in old age. In the elderly the advantages of a single daily injection outweigh those of twice daily injections, such as are usually given to young diabetics. Protamine zinc insulin is the most satisfactory. It should be begun in small doses, of 12—16 units each morning, increasing by 4 units every 3—4 days until glycosuria is abolished. The hazards of nocturnal hypoglycaemia must be guarded against by an adequate evening meal. If the dose of PZ1 reaches 36—40 units, soluble insulin is then begun as a single combined injection, and increments of 4 units every 3—4 days continued. In this way an individualized dose is achieved.

Local skin reactions to insulin are not unduly common in the elderly, and may be expected to disappear in 2—4 weeks (Malins, 1968).

Management of Diabetes During Acute Illness and Surgical Operations

The principles of management of diabetes during acute illnesses in the elderly, and during and after surgical operations, do not differ from those applicable to the young and middle-aged. During acute infections, the diabetic state may worsen, or reduction in food intake may result in hypoglycaemia if the patient is on insulin or an hypoglycaemic agent. Frequent urine tests are the most satisfactory practical method of deciding what is happening. If there is persistent glycosuria or hyperglycaemia, frequent small doses of soluble insulin should be given. No reliance should ever be placed on oral hypoglycaemic agents (Malins, 1968). If there is no glycosuria or hyperglycaemia, no action is required until food intake is resumed. These elementary principles should be known to those caring for elderly people whether at home or in an institution. Any absolute rules — such as that during acute illness, insulin or oral hypoglycaemic agents should *always* be stopped, or the dose *always* increased — are dangerous.

The control of diabetes during and after surgical operations in the elderly is best carried out by a physician with an interest in diabetes.

Patients on diet alone require no particular action before or during surgical operations, except for regular urine testing in the immediate postoperative phase and small doses of soluble insulin if there is hyperglycaemia or glycosuria. Oral hypoglycaemic agents should be discontinued 24—48 hours before operation; management is then as for patients on diet alone. Patients on insulin should receive one-third of their normal daily dose with their premedication, together with intravenous glucose 1 g per unit of insulin. After operation insulin should be given 4—6 hourly according to the urine sugar. The maximum possible dose over 24 hours, with gross glycosuria in all specimens, should approximate to 50 per cent above the patient's usual daily requirements. Hypoglycaemia should always be avoided, and the blood sugar maintained at slightly above normal levels for a few days after operation.

Other Aspects of Management

Regular urine testing is as necessary a part of the management of diabetes in old age as in younger patients. The fact that the renal threshold for glucose rises with age (Butterfield et al., 1967) should not deter from this discipline. Initially daily urine tests are desirable, but once satisfactory control has been established by diet or oral therapy, one or two tests per week, taken after the largest meal of the day, are all that is needed. To test only fasting or early morning specimens is illogical, since they show the situation at its best; sugar-free tests done after meals show that the situation at its worst is satisfactory, and all is thus well.

Many elderly diabetics, particularly those on insulin, benefit from the support and advice provided by regular attendance at a diabetic clinic, but many can be entirely satisfactorily managed by a regular visit from a nurse or health visitor.

MANAGEMENT OF LONG-TERM DIABETES

Diabetics who develop their disease in middle age and survive with it into old age present different problems. Any régime which has proved its value should be left unchanged, and in particular attempts to discontinue insulin therapy of many years duration should be resisted. Oral therapy is almost certain to fail in such patients, and natural complaints of the increasing burden of injections should be met with the advice that what is known to be correct for the individual should not be disturbed.

The main practical difficulties arise from increasing frailty, or the effects of arthritis of the hands, or visual or mental impairment. It should be almost always possible to arrange for injections to be given by a member of the family after instruction by a nurse. Only those with severe visual impairment who live alone should require daily visits from a nurse to give insulin, and institutional care should never be necessary solely so that insulin injections can be given. Changes of diet are relatively rarely necessary, but if the calorie intake seems excessive, review of the diet and perhaps a reduction in intake, accompanied by a reduction in insulin dose, may be desirable. The essential principle is to remember the wise advice: 'Don't try to teach old diabetic dogs new tricks'.

DISORDERED DIABETES
Diabetic Ketosis

Between 12 and 20 per cent of all cases of diabetic ketosis occur in patients over the age of 60 (Barnett et al., 1962; Malins, 1968; Campbell et al., 1973). In the majority, ketosis is precipitated by infection; omission of insulin and diabetes presenting with ketosis are less common in old age, but multiple causes are not infrequent. Much can be done to prevent ketosis by close attention to the diabetic state during acute infections. The infection can be in almost any site, but urinary tract infection and pulmonary tuberculosis (Malins, 1968) should always be remembered, and excluded before the patient leaves hospital.

The clinical features of ketosis in the elderly are essentially the same as those in younger patients, with thirst and polyuria, vomiting and confusion predominating as presenting symptoms (Campbell et al., 1973). As measured by the mean blood glucose on admission, the severity of the metabolic decompensation is if anything greater in the elderly than in younger patients (Barnett et al., 1962); Campbell et al. (1973) report a mean blood sugar of 636 mg/100 ml (40 mmol/l) with a range of 300–1200 mg/100 ml (19–75 mmol/l). The serum osmolarity is commonly raised and tends to increase with increasing degrees of hyperglycaemia, in association with increasing degrees of impairment of consciousness. The serum sodium may vary from hypo- to hypernatraemic levels, and the serum potassium may similarly be high or low. The serum bicarbonate is reduced and blood urea usually raised.

The principles of treatment of diabetic ketosis are the same at any age and are determined by the individual clinical state, in particular the evidence of volume depletion, the precipitating cause, and the biochemical findings. Patients without substantial degrees of hyperosmolarity are best treated with normal saline, followed by hypotonic dextrose solutions with added potassium when the blood sugar fails; and those with hyperosmolarity are best treated with hypotonic solutions throughout. The mean fluid intake in the first 24 hours averages 6–7 litres. In most reported series upwards of 800 units of soluble insulin are given in the first 24 hours. The initial doses are given intravenously. Repeated biochemical estimations are necessary, their frequency depending on the patient's clinical condition and the rate of change of the biochemical disturbance.

Diabetic ketosis in an elderly patient is a serious condition, the mortality in patients over 60 varying from 12 per cent (Barnett et al., 1962) to 30 per cent (Fitzgerald et al., 1961), or at least 3–4 times that of younger patients. Some die within the first 24 hours from the effects of ketosis itself, but much of the mortality is due to arterial occlusions in a variety of sites, occurring after recovery from ketosis (Fitzgerald et al., 1961). The combination of myocardial infarction and diabetic ketosis carries a very high mortality at any age (Bradley and Bryfogle, 1956).

Hyperosmolar Non-ketotic Coma

This interesting condition has been increasingly recognized in the past 20 years, and is most common in the elderly (Arieff and Carroll, 1972). A separation from ketotic coma (in which hyperosmolarity is also present) is not strictly possible (Campbell et al., 1974), but there is much to be said on practical grounds for maintaining the distinction. Some 5 per cent of all cases of severe metabolic decompensation in diabetes take this form (Biegelman, 1971; Campbell et al., 1974).

By comparison with ketosis, precipitation by infection is perhaps less common, and a greater proportion of cases have previously undiscovered diabetes. The history of thirst and polyuria covers many days or weeks, and impairment of consciousness develops more slowly, over 2–3 days. Focal neurological signs, including extensor plantar responses, are common, and fits, often focal, are said to occur in a quarter of cases (Askenasy et al., 1977). Hypotension is frequent, but hyperventilation and acetone in the breath are absent (by definition). The principal biochemical findings include a very high blood sugar, hypernatraemia and hyperchloraemia, a normal or raised serum bicarbonate, and a raised blood urea (Nabarro, 1975).

These patients have a very gross water deficit, and despite the raised serum sodium concentration, considerable sodium depletion as well. Their requirements for fluid replacement are greater than those of ketotic patients, and average 8 litres or more in the first 24 hours (Campbell et al., 1974); this should be given in hypotonic form. Most authors find large doses of insulin necessary (Campbell et al., 1974). Fear of serious blood-CSF osmotic disequilibrium is unwarranted (Arieff and Carroll, 1972).

Improvement with treatment is slower than in ketosis and impairment of consciousness may persist for 24 to 48 hours with eventual full recovery; in ketosis such delay would indicate inadequate therapy and a fatal outcome. The mortality of hyperosmolar coma is considerable, death rates of 40–50 per cent being reported (Arieff and Carroll, 1972), but more recently Campbell et al. (1974) report only 2 deaths in 11 consecutive cases. As in ketosis, many deaths are due to arterial occlusions (Halmos et al., 1966; and others).

Lactic Acidosis

This may complicate a major illness such as myocardial infarction, massive pulmonary embolism or diabetic ketosis which results in poor tissue perfusion, with consequent increased tissue production and decreased hepatic utilization of lactate, or be due to phenformin therapy (Alberti and Nattrass, 1977). Correction of the circulatory defect and alkali therapy constitute the main lines of treatment, but in the elderly this under-recognized condition is likely to have a very high mortality.

Hypoglycaemia

Hypoglycaemia is a manifestation of badly controlled diabetes, and is particularly important in the elderly because it is so dangerous. Prolonged hypoglycaemia at any age can result in irreversible brain damage, but this is certainly considerably more common in the elderly. The manifestations of hypoglycaemia are essentially the same at any age and consist of the acute onset of cerebral symptoms, shown either as diffuse brain dysfunction, with a confusional state progressing to stupor and coma, or, as is particularly important in the elderly, focal cerebral dysfunction, with hemiparesis or on occasions, brain-stem disorder. Meyer et al. (1954) showed in monkeys that the combination of a local arterial lesion and a reduction in blood glucose concentration could produce a hemiplegia; the same is undoubtedly true in man. It follows that when an elderly diabetic on insulin or an oral hypoglycaemic agent develops an acute neuro-psychiatric disorder, with a confusional state or a hemiplegia, whether or not accompanied by the extracerebral manifestations of hypoglycaemia such as sweating, tachycardia and raised blood pressure, hypoglycaemia must be the initial working diagnosis. Blood should be taken for blood sugar estimation, and the blood sugar should be raised forthwith, either by oral administration of glucose if the patient can swallow, or with intravenous glucose if he cannot. If the cerebral state returns to normal within a few minutes, then there is no need for the blood sugar to be estimated. If it does not, then either intractable hypoglycaemia is present, or the neuropsychiatric disorder has some other cause.

Chronic mild hypoglycaemia with impairment of intellectual function persisting over a period of days or even weeks may present particular problems in diagnosis, particularly if the diabetic state is thought to be under good control because there is no glycosuria. Under these circumstances again the blood sugar should be measured, and if, as is usually the case, an oral hypoglycaemic agent is being given, this must be stopped at once, and an adequate glucose intake ensured.

Once the diagnosis of hypoglycaemia has been made it is essential to establish the cause of the particular episode under consideration and remedy it. This is likely to be one of three:

1. Interruption of food intake: the hypoglycaemia will not recur so long as adequate food intake is maintained.

2. Excessive exercise (rare in the elderly): increased glucose intake is necessary.

3. No apparent cause: the dose of insulin or oral agent should be reduced.

CONTROL OF DIABETES AND DEVELOPMENT OF COMPLICATIONS

That there is a relationship between control of diabetes and the development of its specific microvascular complications in the eye and kidney has long been an article of faith among many physicians interested in diabetes (Marble, 1966), and equally fervently disbelieved by others (Bondy, 1966). In recent years it has become increasingly difficult to ignore the weight of acceptable factual evidence in favour of such a relationship. To reviews of this evidence in respect of retinopathy (Caird et al., 1969; Caird, 1971) have been added further clinical data (Pirart, 1977); and, perhaps more important because more likely to convince sceptics, clear demonstrations of the effect of control of experimental diabetes in animals on the development of retinopathy in the diabetic dog (Engerman et al., 1977) and of glomerular lesions in the diabetic rat (Fox et al., 1977). It does not of course follow that because good control reduces the frequency of microvascular lesions in young and middle-aged diabetics that it also does so in old age, but it has been possible to show that this is in fact the case, and that control during the first few years of diagnosed diabetes may be as important in preventing complications in the elderly as in younger diabetics (Caird et al., 1969). It is also probable, though less certainly demonstrated, that good control retards the progression of established retinopathy (Kohner et al., 1969; Miki et al., 1969). It would seem reasonable to conclude that as in younger patients one major reason for attempting to achieve good control of diabetes in old age is to reduce the risk of microvascular complications, but that good control cannot be relied on to prevent progression of established lesions.

There is also evidence, if less satisfactory than for retinopathy, that better controlled older diabetics may have a lesser risk of development of lens opacities (Burditt et al., 1968); again, progression of established opacities does not appear to be affected.

Table 13.1. Deaths by age from circulatory disorders (ICD 400–468) in diabetes (from Hayward and Lucena, 1965)

	Women			Men		
Age	Actual	Expected	Actual/ Expected %	Actual	Expected	Actual/ Expected %
40–49	1	1·1	91	10	2·1	524
50–59	43	9·7	442	19	10·5	180
60–69	104	48·6	214	58	30·8	188
70–79	144	88·6	162	50	40	125
80 +	29	30·6	95	24	17·4	138

The situation with regard to atherosclerotic disease of large vessels is more confused. There is a substantial excess mortality among diabetics from circulatory disorders (*Table* 13.1); this is apparent at all ages in men and up to the age of 80 in women. There is no doubt from epidemiological studies that diabetes is an important risk factor for such disease in all three of its major sites — heart, leg and brain (Keen et al., 1965; Kingsbury, 1966; Epstein, 1967). Data from the Framingham study show this to be the case in the elderly (Kannel, 1976; *Table* 13.2). The presence of glucose intolerance, compared with its absence, is associated with a two- to three-fold increase in the risk of the development of intermittent claudication, hypertensive heart failure and 'atherothrombotic brain infarction'. Smoking is more important in respect of intermittent claudication; blood pressure in respect of stroke; and blood pressure and abnormality of the electro-cardiogram equally important in respect of hypertensive heart failure; but

Table 13.2. Approximate 'multipliers' for various risk factors for vascular disease in elderly men (*see text*; after Kannel, 1976)

		Hypertensive heart failure	Intermittent claudication	Atherothrombotic brain infarction
Age	Years	70	70	65
Duration of follow-up	Years	18	18	8
Glucose intolerance	Yes *vs* No	3·0	2·5	2·0
Smoking	Yes *vs* No	1·5	3·0	2·0
Left ventricular hypertrophy*	Yes *vs* No	3·0	2·0	1·25
Systolic blood pressure	195 *vs* 150 mmHg	3·0	1·5	3·0
Serum cholesterol	335 *vs* 260 mg/100ml	1·1	1·25	1·0

* On ECG.

glucose intolerance is more important in respect of all three than is hyper-cholesterolaemia. There can thus be little doubt about the significance of the relationship.

There is however much greater uncertainty about any possible associa-tion between control of diabetes and the subsequent development of clinically apparent arterial disease at any age. The problem is further complicated by the finding of the University Diabetes Group Program (1970) that the treatment of diabetes with sulphonylureas, and perhaps also biguanides (Knatterud et al., 1971), may be associated with an increased mortality from myocardial infarction. This study has been severely criti-cized on methodological grounds (Editorial *Lancet*, 1971; Seltzer, 1972), and its findings have not been confirmed elsewhere (Paasakivi, 1970; Keen, 1971). Most British physicians would undoubtedly agree with Lister (1972) that 'the use of oral drugs is justified in patients following a diet and not yet adequately controlled, especially if they are elderly . . .'

COMPLICATIONS OF DIABETES
Ocular Complications
The ocular complications of diabetes are important in old age, both because they may lead to the diagnosis of the metabolic disorder and as a

common cause of visual impairment and blindness. One patient in eight whose diabetes is discovered over the age of 70 presents with an ocular complaint, most often cataract (Caird et al., 1969). The routine testing of urine of elderly patients in ophthalmological clinics is thus a worthwhile procedure (McIlwaine and Smith, 1966; Caird et al., 1969). In addition, 20 per cent of elderly diabetics at the time of diagnosis of diabetes show refractive changes (usually increased myopia), while 12 per cent have evidence of retinopathy (Soler et al., 1969).

Over the age of 70, 7 per cent of newly registered blindness is due to diabetic retinopathy (Sorsby, 1966), and because diabetics are not immune to non-diabetic ocular disorders, as many as 10 per cent of the elderly blind are diabetics (Caird et al., 1969). The incidence of blindness due to retinopathy over the age of 70 is 20 times that between the ages of 30 and 50, and the prevalence about 10 times greater. Figures such as these are evidence of the great importance of diabetes as a cause of blindness in old age.

About 40 per cent of all diabetics over the age of 60 show evidence of retinopathy (Caird et al., 1969). This is usually of so-called 'background' type, with microaneurysms, occasional haemorrhages and especially hard exudates, which are often circinate in pattern, lying in a ring around the macula. Involvement of the macula itself leads to serious impairment of vision. Proliferative retinopathy, with new vessel formation and preretinal haemorrhage, is relatively rare in old age. Yet despite the rarity of this sinister variety of retinopathy, prognosis for vision is worse the older the patient. In older diabetics with background retinopathy, 38 per cent of those with initial good vision have a visual acuity of 6/18 or less in the better eye after 5 years, and 20 per cent an acuity of less than 6/60 (Caird et al., 1968). There is little evidence that meticulous control of diabetes greatly improves the prognosis of established retinopathy in the elderly diabetic, but photocoagulation has been clearly shown to benefit macular disease (Multicentre Study Group, 1975), and clofibrate increases the rate of disappearance of hard exudates (Cullen et al., 1964), though often with little improvement in vision (Harrold et al., 1969).

The second major ocular complication of diabetes is cataract. The epidemiological evidence on the controversial question of the relative frequency of cataract in diabetics and non-diabetics may be summarized as follows (Caird, 1973): lens opacities are no commoner in older diabetics than non-diabetics, but cataract extraction is 3—4 times commoner, and it must thus be presumed that the rate of advance of lens opacities and maturation of cataract is more rapid in diabetics. Both lens opacities and cataract extraction are commoner in diabetic women than men (Burditt et al., 1968).

The clinical appearances of cataract in elderly diabetics are identical to those of non-diabetic senile cataract, and the indications for operation are the same (Caird et al., 1969). The presence of diabetes should never deter or delay the decision to operate if this is indicated. The management of diabetes before and after operation should be in the hands of a physician experienced in diabetes, but extremely precise control of diabetes should not be regarded as a necessity as there is no good evidence that minor degrees of hyperglycaemia affect the outcome (Owens and Hughes, 1947). No particular operative technique is usually advised in diabetics. Complications of cataract extraction are little commoner in diabetics than non-diabetics, except for capsular rupture (Ramsell, 1970), and perhaps iritis (Caird et al., 1969). In the absence of retinopathy the visual results are identical, 80 per cent having a good result (visual acuity 6/12 or better) and 5–10 per cent a poor result (visual less than 6/60). If there is retinopathy, only one-third achieve a good result, and one-third have a poor result (Caird et al., 1969). However, even in the presence of quite severe retinopathy, and when there is no great improvement of visual acuity, an elderly diabetic may gain a truly worthwhile result from operation.

Diabetic ophthalmoplegia is best regarded as a true ischaemic neuropathy and is described below (p. 174). The ophthalmoscopically alarming conditions of asteroid hyalitis and synchisis scintillans are occasionally seen in elderly diabetics: the former should not be confused with retinal exudates, while the latter is a spectacular curiosity; neither affects vision.

Renal Disease

The complex combination of pathological processes which goes by the name of diabetic nephropathy has been reviewed by Thomsen (1965) and Cameron et al. (1975). All the characteristic lesions (thickening of glomerular capillary basement membranes, accumulation of basement membrane substance in the mesangium and as nodules in the capillary loops, and arteriolar lesions) occur in the elderly, and indeed the original description of the nodular lesions by Kimmelstiel and Wilson (1936) included several elderly patients.

Nephropathy increases in frequency with increasing duration of diabetes, but may be diagnosed at or soon after the diagnosis of diabetes in old age (O'Sullivan, 1961), exactly as with retinopathy. The principal clinical manifestation is proteinuria, but this may only be present when there is much glomerular damage (Gellman et al., 1959), and is in any case not specific for nephropathy. Oedema is not unusual, but a true nephrotic syndrome with hypoalbuminaemia is rare. The blood pressure is rarely greatly raised. At least 80 per cent show diabetic retinopathy. Gross impairment of renal function is unusual and progression is on average slow (Watkins et al., 1972). The survival rate of diabetics with proteinuria is about half that of all diabetics (Caird, 1961). Death from renal failure is less common than from coexisting coronary artery disease.

Urinary tract infection as manifest by bacteriuria is not more frequent in elderly diabetics than in non-diabetics (O'Sullivan et al., 1961). When diagnosed it should be treated in the usual way. One relatively rare complication of renal infection is however particularly common in diabetics. About 50 per cent of cases of renal papillary necrosis are diabetics (Lauler et al., 1960). The clinical manifestations vary from the trivial, so that it presents as an unexpected autopsy finding, to a very severe acute pyelonephritis with pain, high fever and often substantial reduction in renal function. A subsequent intravenous pyelogram may show loss of papillae.

Neurological Disorders

The neurological complications of diabetes contribute substantially to disability in elderly diabetics, because diabetic neuropathy is an important cause of lesions of the feet (*see below*) and diabetic amyotrophy an important problem in its own right. Classification of the neurological complications of diabetes is very difficult (Malins, 1968), and recent reviews (Colby, 1965; Thomas and Ward, 1975) have concentrated on a simple distinction between a symmetrical, largely sensory, subacute or chronic polyneuropathy with a generally poor prognosis (diabetic neuropathy), and a group of asymmetrical, largely motor, often painful, acute conditions, with a relatively good prognosis. It is clear that both types of condition may coexist, and neuropathologists find it difficult to make any clear distinction between them (Greenbaum, 1964). Involvement of the autonomic nervous system creates a third group of disorders.

Table 13.3. Signs suggestive of neuropathy in diabetics and non-diabetics (Mayne, 1965)

	Number examined		Percentage with absent or impaired:						
			Knee jerk		Ankle jerk		Vibration sense		Position sense	
Diabetes	−	+	−	+	−	+	−	+	−	+
Age										
0−29	8	16	0	31	0	44	25	6	0	19
30−49	25	44	10	40	5	61	0	30	10	19
50−69	57	109	11	24	33	83	16	59	36	41
70 +	25	50	16	42	40	84	67	85	52	68

1. Sensory Polyneuropathy

Symmetrical sensory polyneuropathy is usually a complication of long-standing diabetes, and in the elderly may be difficult to diagnose with confidence, because of the high frequency of abnormal signs in elderly subjects without diabetes (Mayne, 1965). Nevertheless, elderly diabetics show such signs more frequently than non-diabetics (*Table* 13.3). Loss of light touch and pain sense should be regarded as evidence of a significant neuropathy. The sensory loss in the feet is often implicated in the genesis of perforating ulceration of the feet, with osteitis and abscess formation in the foot (Oakley et al., 1956). Nocturnal pain and calf tenderness are unusual in elderly diabetics with neuropathy. The management of this type of neuropathy in old age consists in protection of the feet from ill-fitting shoes and other sources of trauma.

2. *Diabetic Amyotrophy*

The less common condition of diabetic amyotrophy (Garland, 1955; Locke et al., 1963) requires to be recognized because of its different prognosis, and to avoid unnecessary investigation. Characteristically, an elderly patient, often with no previous history of diabetes, develops over a period of weeks or months pain, weakness and wasting, first in one thigh, and then the other; difficulty in walking may be gross. Sensory loss may be absent, and reflex changes reflect muscle wasting. The plantar responses may be, or become, extensor. Nerve conduction studies show diminished conduction velocities in the femoral nerve, and muscle biopsy may show disseminated atrophy of single muscle fibres, unlike that encountered in lesions of the anterior horn cell or nerve root (Locke et al., 1963).

The condition usually progresses for some weeks or months, remains static for a further period of months, and then slowly improves, with usually complete and permanent recovery of motor power (but not of sensory loss if present) in 12—18 months (Casey and Harrison, 1972). Although this natural course may occur without particular attention to control of the diabetes, most physicians would regard diabetic amyotrophy as an important indication for strict control, as this seems likely to accelerate recovery.

3. *Diabetic Ophthalmoplegia*

It is doubtful if other mononeuropathies are truly commoner in diabetics than non-diabetics, apart from diabetic ophthalmoplegia. In this condition (Zorilla and Kozak, 1967), which usually affects the elderly diabetic, there is a period of unilateral headache, followed by the development of a third or sixth nerve palsy. If the third nerve is involved, there is characteristically sparing of the pupil (Goldstein and Cogan, 1960), probably because the lesion is vascular and affects the centre of the nerve, while the pupillomotor fibres run in the periphery (Sunderland and Hughes, 1946). In typical cases investigation for intracranial aneurysm or other sinister cause can be avoided. The ophthalmoplegia recovers in 3—6 months.

4. *Autonomic Neuropathy*

Diabetic autonomic neuropathy is a further group of conditions not infrequently encountered in old age. Other evidence of somatic neuropathy is usually present, but the duration of diabetes varies greatly. Three syndromes are of importance:

a. Postural Hypotension. Postural hypotension is due to afferent dener-
vation of the baroreceptor reflexes (Sharpey-Shafer and Taylor, 1960).
Syncopal episodes on standing must be distinguished from hypoglycaemic
attacks and the diagnosis confirmed by the recording of the blood pressure
in the standing as well as the lying position. The heart rate is usually
fixed and does not rise on standing nor change on deep breathing (Wheeler
and Watkins, 1973). Firm full length elastic stockings, and if necessary
fludrocortisone 0·1—0·3 mg/d, will assist in controlling this troublesome
condition (Johnson, 1976).

b. Diabetic Diarrhoea. Episodic or continuous diarrhoea, often preceded
by loud borborygmi and accompanied by noctural incontinence of faeces,
is characteristic of diabetic diarrhoea (Malins and French, 1957). Nutrition
is well preserved, since there is no malabsorption. There is usually evidence
of symmetrical neuropathy and often retinopathy and proteinuria. Barium
enema and sigmoidoscopy are normal. The recognition of this most dis-
tressing condition is important because the majority of cases respond to
antibiotic treatment with tetracycline (Malins and French, 1957); the
addition of metronidazole may well be helpful. The presumed mechanism
of the diarrhoea is bacterial colonization of the small bowel.

c. Bladder Disorder. In this condition, whose frequency is probably considerably underestimated, there is a dilated atonic bladder with the eventual
development of overflow retention. Ellenberg (1966) described 27 cases,
of whom 17 were over 60 years of age, and stressed the importance of
factors leading to immobility (e.g. surgical operations and major fractures)
in precipitating retention. Most patients have evidence of somatic neuropathy. Cystometry shows a large residual urine, a long low pressure curve
on filling and lack of bladder sensation. Temporary catheterization and
treatment of any urinary infection present often result in functional
improvement, but surgical treatment by bladder neck resection may be
necessary and is usually highly effective.

Vascular Disease
The principal problem of diagnosis of ischaemic heart disease in the
elderly diabetic is the presentation of myocardial infarction as disordered
diabetes. The mortality of myocardial infarction in elderly diabetics is
high, particularly in women who have been on oral hypoglycaemic therapy
(Soler et al., 1975), and if frank ketosis is present (Bradley and Bryfogle,
1956). The urgent necessity to exclude hypoglycaemia in a diabetic on
insulin or oral therapy who presents with the sudden onset of focal neurological signs has been mentioned (p. 168); the management of elderly
diabetics with stroke does not otherwise differ from that of non-diabetics.

The Diabetic Foot
Lesions of the feet in elderly diabetics constitute a most important cause
of morbidity and of prolonged admission to hospital. As in younger

patients, three elements — ischaemia, neuropathy, and sepsis — singly or in combination, are involved in the genesis of foot lesions and accurate assessment of the contribution of each is essential for proper management (Oakley et al., 1956; Catterall, 1972).

Ischaemic lesions include both massive gangrene from major arterial occlusion and gangrene of individual toes from pressure or trauma. Presence of foot pulses virtually excludes an ischaemic origin, but the pulses may be impossible to feel in a swollen but non-ischaemic foot. A cold foot with atrophic hairless skin, and a temperature gradient at some point in the calf, is ischaemic.

Two common neuropathic lesions are encountered: blisters on the toes which rupture to leave superficial gangrenous patches and shallow granulating ulcers, and ulceration below the first metatarsophalangeal joint, often with extension into the joint, and sometimes abscess formation in the sole. The foot will be warm, and the pulses usually palpable. The septic lesions may complicate either ischaemia or neuropathy. X-rays of the feet may show extensive bone destruction in neuropathic-septic lesions; calcification in the dorsalis pedis artery should be ignored.

Preventive measures pay major invisible dividends: simple foot hygiene, proper footwear, avoidance of damaging extremes of heat and cold and regular attendance at a chiropodist. Neuropathic blisters will heal with rest and antibiotics, but bone necrosis and abscess formation require surgical treatment, usually amputation of a toe or metatarsal (ray amputation) and drainage of an abscess. Considerable surgical judgement is needed to decide the best course of conservative or radical treatment of ischaemic lesions. Amputation of a toe often fails to result in healing (Malins, 1968), and a prolonged period in hospital may follow even a minor amputation. But the late mortality of patients who require a high amputation is considerable (Cameron et. al., 1964; Whitehouse et al., 1968). Much of this mortality is due to coexisting coronary artery disease (Malins, 1968). As many as a quarter of patients come to a second amputation before they die.

Infections

The frequency of pulmonary tuberculosis in diabetics is undoubtedly much less than before the introduction of chemotherapy (Malins, 1968), but there can be no doubt of an excess prevalence among diabetics at all ages (Oscarsson and Silwer, 1958). It remains reasonable to carry out a chest radiograph on every newly discovered elderly diabetic, and on all diabetics admitted to hospital. Tuberculosis may precipitate ketosis in the elderly, and no elderly patient should be allowed to leave hospital after an episode of ketosis without a chest X-ray.

Skin infections are traditionally commoner in diabetics, but severe infections such as carbuncles are now rare. Antibiotic therapy and surgical drainage if necessary, combined with control of the likely accompanying disordered diabetes, is highly effective.

REFERENCES

Alberti K. G. M. M. and Nattrass M. (1977) *Lancet* 2, 25.

Alexander W. D. and Marples J. (1977) *Lancet* 1, 191.

Arieff A. I. and Carroll H. J. (1972) *Medicine (Baltimore)* 51, 73.

Askenasy J. J., Streifler M. and Carosso R. (1977) *Eur. Neurol.* 16, 51.

Balodimos M. C., Camerini-Davalos R. A. and Marble A. (1966) *Metabolism* 16, 957.

Barnett D. M., Wilcox D. S. and Marble A. (1962) *Geriatrics* 17, 327.

Bergman U., Boman G. and Wiholm B. E. (1978) *Br. Med. J.* 2, 464.

Biegelman P. M. (1971) *Diabetes* 20, 490.

Björntorp P., Carlström S., Fagerberg S. E. et al. (1978) *Diabetologia* 15, 95.

Bloom, A. and Richards J. G. (1961) *Br. Med. J.* 1, 1796.

Bondy P. K. (1966) In: Ingelfinger F. J., Relman A. S. and Finland M. (ed.) *Controversy in Internal Medicine*, Philadelphia, Saunders, p. 499.

Bradley R. D. and Bryfogle J. W. (1956) *Am. J. Med.* 20, 207.

British Diabetic Association (1973) *The Care of the Elderly Diabetic.* London and Tonbridge, Whitefriars.

Burditt A. F., Caird F. I. and Draper G. D. (1968) *Br. J. Ophthalmol.* 52, 433.

Butterfield W. J. H., Keen H. and Whichelow M. J. (1967) *Br. Med. J.* 4, 505.

Caird F. I. (1961) *Diabetes* 10, 178.

Caird F. I. (1973) In: Pirie A. ed. *The Human Lens – in Relation to Cataract. Ciba Foundation Symposium* 19, Amsterdam, Elsevier, p. 281.

Caird F. I. (1971) *Acta Diabetol. Lat.* 8, Suppl. 1, 394.

Caird F. I., Burditt A. F. and Draper G. D. (1968) *Diabetes* 17, 121.

Caird F. I., Pirie A. and Ramsall T. G. (1969) *Diabetes and the Eye.* Oxford and Edinburgh, Blackwell.

Cameron H. C., Lennard-Jones J. E. and Robinson M. P. (1964) *Lancet* 2, 605.

Cameron J. S., Ireland J. T. and Watkins P. J. (1975) In: Keen H. and Jarrett J. (ed.) *Complications of Diabetes.* London, Edward Arnold, p. 99.

Campbell I. W., Munro J. F. and Duncan L. J. P. (1973) *Age Ageing* 2, 199.

Campbell I. W., Munro J. F. and Duncan L. J. P. (1974) *Scott. Med. J.* 19, 177.

Casey E. B. and Harrison M. J. G. (1972) *Br. Med. J.* 1, 656.

Catterall R. C. F. (1972) *Br. J. Hosp. Med.* 7, 224.

Cervantes-Amezcua A., Naldjian S., Camerini-Davalos R. et al. (1965) *J. Am. Med. Assoc.* 193, 759.

Colby A. (1965) *Diabetes* 14, 424 and 516.

Cullen J. F., Ireland J. T. and Oliver M. F. (1964) *Trans. Ophthalmol. Soc. UK* 84, 281.

de Troyer A. and Demanet J. C. (1976) *Q. J. Med.* 45, 52.

DHSS (1972) 3 (*see* General References).

Editorial (1971) *Lancet* 1, 171.

Ellenberg M. (1966) *Arch. Intern. Med.* 117, 348.

Engerman R., Bloodworth J. M. B. and Nelson S. (1977) *Diabetes* 26, 760.

Epstein F. H. (1967) *Circulation* 36, 609.

Fitzgerald M. G., O'Sullivan D. J. and Malins J. M. (1961) *Br. Med. J.* 1, 247.

Fox C. J., Darby S. C., Ireland J. T. et al. (1977) *Br. Med. J.* 2, 605.

Gale E. A. M. and Tattersall R. B. (1976) *Br. Med. J.* 2, 972.

Garcia M., Miller M. and Moses M. (1971) *Ann. Intern. Med.* 75, 549.

Garland H. (1955) *Br. Med. J.* 2, 1287.

Gellman D. D., Pirani C. L., Soothill J. F. et al. (1959) *Medicine (Baltimore)* 38, 321.

Goldstein J. E. and Cogan D. G. (1960) *Arch. Ophthalmol.* 64, 592.

Greenbaum D. (1964) *Brain* 87, 215.

Halmos P. B., Nelson J. K. and Lowry R. C. (1966) *Lancet* 1, 675.

Harrold B. P., Marmion V. J. and Gough K. R. (1969) *Diabetes* 18, 285.

Hayward R. E. and Lucena B. C. (1965) *J. Inst. Actuaries* 91, 286.

Johnson R. H. (1976) In: Caird F. I., Dall J. L. C. and Kennedy R. D. (ed.), *Cardiology in Old Age.* New York and London, Plenum, p. 101.

Kannel W. B. (1976) In: Caird F. I., Dall J. L. C. and Kennedy R. D. (ed.), *Cardiology in Old Age*. New York and London, Plenum, p. 143.
Keen H. (1971) *Acta Diabetol. Lat.* 8, Suppl. 1, 444.
Keen H., Rose G. A., Pyke D. A. et al. (1965) *Lancet* 2, 505.
Kimmelstiel P. and Wilson C. (1936) *Am. J. Pathol.* 12, 83.
Kingsbury K. J. (1966) *Lancet* 2, 1374.
Knatterud G. L., Meinert C. T., Klimt C. R. et al. (1971) *J. Am. Med. Assoc.* 217, 777.
Kohner E., Fraser T. R., Joplin G. F. et al. (1969) In: Goldberg M. F. and Fine S. L. (ed.), *Symposium on the Treatment of Diabetic Retinopathy*. Washington DC, US Public Health Service Publ. No. 190, p. 119.
Lauler D. P., Schreiner G. E. and David A. (1960) *Am. J. Med.* 29, 132.
Lister J. (1972) *Br. J. Hosp. Med.* 7, 171.
Locke S., Lawrence D. G. and Legge M. A. (1963) *Am. J. Med.* 34, 775.
McIlwaine C. L. K. and Smith A. W. M. (1966) *Scott. Med. J.* 11, 208.
MacLeod C. C. (1970) *Nutrition (London)* 24, 24.
MacLeod C. C. and Caird F. I. (1975) *Nutrition (London)* 29, 153.
MacLeod C. C., Judge T. G. and Caird F. I. (1974) *Age Ageing* 3, 158.
Malins J. (1968) *Clinical Diabetes Mellitus*. London, Eyre & Spottiswoode.
Malins J. M. and French J. M. (1957) *Q. J. Med.* 26, 467.
Marble A. (1966) In: Ingelfinger F. J., Relman A. S. and Finland M. (ed.), *Controversy in Internal Medicine*. Philadelphia, Saunders, p. 491.
Mayne N. M. (1965) *Lancet* 2, 1313.
Meyer J. F., Fang H. C. and Denny-Brown D. (1954) *Arch. Neurol. Psychiatr.* 72, 296.
Miki E., Fukuda M., Kuzuya T. et al. (1969) *Diabetes* 18, 773.
Multicentre Study Group (1975) *Lancet* 2, 1110.
Nabarro J. D. N. (1975) In: Leibel B. S. and Wrenshall G. A. (ed.) *On the Nature and Treatment of Diabetes. International Congress Series No. 84*. The Hague, Excerpta Medica, p. 545.
Oakley W. G., Catterall R. C. F. and Martin M. M. (1956) *Br. Med. J.* 2, 953.
Oscarsson P. N. and Silwer H. (1958) *Acta Med. Scand.* 161, Suppl. 335, 23.
O'Sullivan D. J. (1961) Cited by Malins (1968).
O'Sullivan D. J., Fitzgerald M. G., Meynell M. J. et al. (1961) *Br. Med. J.* 1, 786.
Owens W. C. and Hughes W. F. (1947) *Arch. Ophthalmol.* 37, 561.
Paasakivi J. (1970) *Acta Med. Scand.* 187, Suppl. 507, 9.
Patel D. P. and Stowers J. M. (1964) *Lancet* 2, 282.
Pirart J. (1977) *Diabete et Metabolisme (Paris)* 3, 97, 173 and 245.
Ramsell T. G. (1970) *Acta Diabetol. Lat.* 7, 789.
Schen R. J. and Benaroya Y. (1976) *Age Ageing* 5, 31.
Seltzer H. S. (1972) *Diabetes* 21, 976.
Sharpey-Shafer E. P. and Taylor P. J. (1960) *Lancet* 1, 559.
Soler N. G., Bennett M. A., Pentecost B. L. et al. (1975) *Q. J. Med.* 44, 125.
Soler N. G., Fitzgerald M. G., Malins J. M. et al. (1969) *Br. Med. J.* 3, 567.
Sorsby A. (1966) DHSS Report Public Health and Medical Subjects No. 114, London, HMSO.
Sunderland S., and Hughes E. S. R. (1946) *Brain* 69, 301.
Thomas B. J. Truswell A. S. and Brown A. M. (1974) *Nutrition (London)* 28, 297.
Thomas P. K. and Ward J. D. (1975) In: Keen H. and Jarrett J. (ed.), *Complications of Diabetes*. London, Edward Arnold, p. 151.
Thomsen A. C. (1965) *The Kidney in Diabetes Mellitus*. Copenhagen, Munksgaard.
Tunbridge R. and Wetherill J. H. (1970) *Br. Med. J.* 2, 78.
University Diabetes Group Program (1970) *Diabetes* 19, Suppl. 2, 747.
Watkins P. J., Blainey J. D., Brewer D. B. et al. (1972) *Q. J. Med.* 41, 437.

Wheeler T. and Watkins P. J. (1973) *Br. Med. J.* **4**, 584.
Whitehouse F. W., Jurgensen C. and Block M. A. (1968) *Diabetes* **17**, 520.
Wise P. H., Chapman M., Thomas D. W. et al. (1976) *Br. Med. J.* **1**, 70.
Zorilla E. and Kozak G. P. (1967) *Ann. Intern. Med.* **67**, 968.

14. PITUITARY FUNCTION AND DISEASES
M. F. Green

It has often been suggested that a decline in the function of endocrine glands and in their capacity to respond to stress is a cause of senescence or ageing, but there have been few reports of clinical malfunction of the pituitary in old age (Zerny, 1957; Ngu and Paley, 1968; Coni, 1973). Soffer (1951) found no cases of Simmonds's disease starting after the age of 70 but Berthaux et al. (1962) described two patients of 83 and 84 who died in hypopituitary coma. Some patients may now survive into old age with treated pituitary deficiency.

Anterior pituitary gonadotrophins continue to be released at a higher level than previously for many years after their target organs – the ovary and testis – fail. Relatively scanty histopathological evidence has shown age-related changes in the pituitary, but these are inconstant and of doubtful clinical significance, the relationship between pituitary abnormalities found in aged animals and pituitary function in elderly humans is far from clear. Nevertheless, for several reasons, it seems very likely that hypothalamic-pituitary disorders should occur and have been underdiagnosed in the elderly.

There has been little investigation of the elderly by endocrinologists and histopathologists using the latest techniques to test hypothalamic-pituitary and target organ function, or to measure neurotransmitters. What little work there is mainly concerns (a) the pituitary-thyroid axis, using thyrotropin-releasing hormone (TRH) and thyroid-stimulating hormone (TSH) assays; (b) the examination of cortical and subcortical tissues in chronic brain failure (dementia); and (c) the treatment of Parkinsonism with L-dopa and bromocriptine based on neuropharmacological investigation of the basal ganglia. Cerebrovascular and degenerative central nervous system (CNS) diseases are common in old age. The cortical-hypothalamic-pituitary-target organ pathways might sometimes be involved in these pathological processes.

The age-related tendency to develop impairment of autonomic functions which have CNS components, such as temperature control, blood pressure regulation and balance mechanisms might sometimes be due to central abnormalities involving the hypothalamus and pituitary.

The relatively rapid and then long sustained rise of pituitary gonadotrophins after the menopause might sometimes cause the pituitary to become hyperplastic and even autonomously neoplastic, analogous to the mechanism in tertiary hyperparathyroidism. This might also occur in untreated primary hypothyroidism and the pre-hypothyroid state indicated by raised TSH levels; both these situations are found in the aged. Autonomous pituitary abnormalities associated with sustained gonadotrophin and TSH secretion do not seem to have been described.

A rule of geriatric medicine is that extreme old age does not protect from illness. Endocrine disorders can develop insidiously at any age, but it is now well known how serious, but potentially remediable, thyroid disease usually presents in older patients as either a 'failure-to-thrive' syndrome or else in a very modified and atypical form. Almost any endocrinopathy can occur in the elderly. Although diabetes mellitus and thyroid dysfunction are the commonest disorders, it is likely that hypothalamic-pituitary-target organ malfunction is commoner in the elderly than previously recognized. Of course, it is also true that features suggestive of hypothalamic-pituitary-target organ failure may be present but due to other disorders, e.g. hypothermia, hypotension, skin pigmentation etc. Specific endocrine tests should be done where indicated and abnormal results looked at very critically rather than dismissing high or low levels as due to age.

STRUCTURE AND FUNCTION
The hypothalamus is an integral part of the pituitary endocrine factory. *Fig.* 14.1 summarizes the functions and controlling mechanisms of the hypothalamus and anterior pituitary, *Fig.* 14.2 those of the hypothalamus and posterior pituitary. The hypothalamus is directly involved in the feedback mechanisms controlling many pituitary hormones in a whole variety of homeostatic mechanisms (blood pressure, temperature regulation, sleep and metabolism in its broadest sense) which often fail in the elderly.

The hypophysis is supplied by arteries arising from the internal carotid. These might frequently be involved in cerebrovascular disease, and in extracranial vascular problems.

HISTOPATHOLOGY AND HISTOPHYSIOLOGY
The most comprehensive review of the pathology of the aged is by McKeown (1965). She commented that 'diseases of the pituitary are probably the least important of all endocrine disturbances in the aged'. She had found little evidence that the increased number of chromophobe cells and reduction in overall cell numbers and increased interstitial connective tissue which occur with advancing age have any functional implication.

Andrew (1971) has reviewed the findings of a series of authors' observations on ageing of the pituitary in man and animals. Decreased vascularity, increased connective tissue, increased numbers of basophil cells, of con-

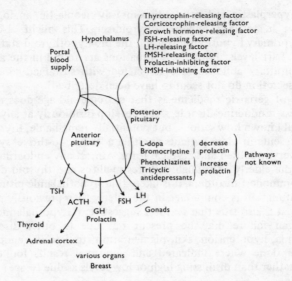

a

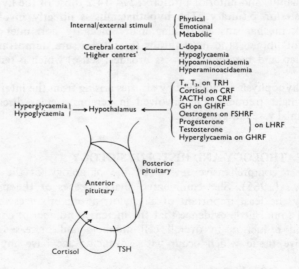

b

Fig. 14.1. *a*, Anterior pituitary hormones. *b*, Control of anterior pituitary.

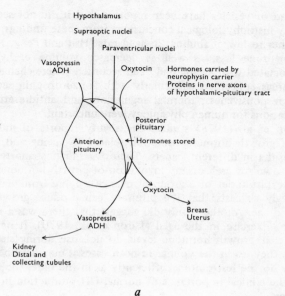

Fig. 14.2. *a*, Posterior pituitary hormones. *b*, Posterior pituitary control.

cretions and of vesicles have been reported, but it did not seem possible to draw any histophysiological conclusions from these findings.

In another review of findings in aged rats (Hsu and Peng, 1978) hypothalamic neurone loss, as well as decreased volume of hypothalamic nuclei, associated with ageing had been recorded. These changes had been noted in areas concerned particularly with gonadotrophin secretion and oestrogen responsiveness, thermal regulation, and antidiuretic response. The implications for human physiology were uncertain.

Calderon et al. (1978) studied the scanty reports of morphological features of growth hormone secretion related to ageing and found very variable results in different papers. There was no post mortem evidence from their own research of any involution of growth hormone producing cells in the pituitaries of a group of over 80s dying from acute illnesses. This strongly suggests that the pituitary can produce growth hormone (GH) in old age. Another study did suggest that there was a reduced GH response to exercise in the aged (Laron et al., 1970). It has also been suggested that growth hormone levels do not rise during sleep in older subjects as they do in the young. In both cases it may have been difficult to actually do the test quite as efficiently as in the older subjects. Unfortunately, the clinical importance of normal GH production in the elderly is not known.

Chromophobe adenomata are the commonest pituitary tumours and have been recorded in elderly people. Five of the 565 patients studied in one series were over the age of 70 (Kernohan and Syare, 1956). These adenomata can cause clinical effects by pressure on neighbouring tissues, such as the optic chiasma, and by destruction of the gland with hypofunction and decline in some or all of the pituitary hormones. The rarer eosinophil adenoma is reported as giving symptoms most often in younger patients. However, the author has seen three acromegalics during the last ten years whose diagnosis was only made in old age, i.e. over 75, although their tumours and abnormal growth production may have started years before. The diagnosis of active disease was confirmed by abnormally raised and non-suppressed growth hormone levels during a glucose tolerance test.

The high incidence of the pituitary tumours found in 1000 glands studied by Costello (1936) and the increasing frequency with advancing age does support the contention that these tumours are under-diagnosed in life. This survey was done a long time ago. The very rapid recent decline in post mortems may be another reason why pituitary disease in old age is hardly ever suspected even in retrospect. Another possibility is that some of these adenomata may not produce significant disease and are non-secretory. Adenomata occur frequently in the prostates of elderly men, but in this organ hypertrophy and carcinoma are diagnosed clinically, although much less frequently than the histopathological changes would imply.

Clinical hyper- and hypopituitarism have rarely been described in old age, apart from a few cases of hyperfunctioning adenomata in younger old patients (i.e. one or two aged about 70 in series with a much younger mean age), or in elderly people being successfully treated for hypofunction after developing this condition as a result of treatment of a hyperfunctioning adenoma.

Of course, even substantial or total pituitary failure in old age would not produce such widespread target organ failure as in younger subjects. Loss of gonadotrophins, growth hormone and oxytocin would not particularly matter. In an 80-year-old hypopituitary man presenting with hypothermia, and successfully treated, it was only necessary to give thyroid and adrenocortical replacement therapy (Exton-Smith, 1972). In passing, it can be commented that the usual aetiology of hypothyroidism in old age is primary failure of the thyroid, due to autoimmune or degenerative disease, or following thyroidectomy or radio-iodine treatment. It is very rare to consider pituitary failure as a cause of hypothyroidism unless symptoms or signs suggest deficiencies in other pituitary target organs. Laboratories may just measure thyroxine (T4), triiodothyronine (T3) uptake or thyroid indices and not carry out routine TSH assays in suspected hypothyroidism. Low TSH levels in conjunction with low thyroid tests would suggest myxoedema secondary to hypopituitarism. It is possible that autoimmune disease could affect the pituitary in old people as this has been described in younger patients (Maisey and Stevens, 1969). This would be somewhat more likely to occur if other autoimmune diseases are present, and of course thyroiditis is thought to be the commonest cause of hypothyroidism in old age.

Many, if not all, of the pituitary hormones work at two levels. They are involved in bodily mechanisms where a basal hormonal output is required to maintain life and normal activity and they are produced at high levels in response to a variety of stresses. In view of the vascular and age-related and senescent histological changes noted in human and animal glands, it is possible that a function of ageing would be to impair or reduce the hypothalamic-pituitary-target organ's functional capacity to stress, whilst retaining the ability to maintain basal hormonal levels. There is no doubt that many old people do succumb more easily to both physical and psychological stresses than younger people. Sometimes this is associated with features which could implicate the pituitary, e.g. hypothermia, lack of pyrexia in infections, hypotension.

However, what dynamic functional testing has been carried out does not support this hypothesis. There is no evidence that general or partial failure of the hypothalamus or pituitary to respond to stress is commonly implicated in disease, or in ageing, in humans.

THE EFFECT OF DRUGS AND DISEASES ON THE PITUITARY
L-dopa can affect pituitary function. Hodkinson (1974) believes that elevated free thyroxine index (FTI) levels in elderly patients receiving

L-dopa are due to a pituitary effect rather than a direct thyroid or protein-binding mechanism. Eddy et al. (1974) have reported that L-dopa suppressed TSH and prolactin, although they did not feel this affected basal thyroid function. They also found that L-dopa affects GH release. TRH given to patients with Parkinson's disease stimulated prolactin release, as well as TSH.

Bigos et al. (1977) have reported a fascinating study of the pathological effects of thyroid failure on the pituitary. There were multiple abnormalities including hyperprolactinaemia, decreased GH secretion and decreased responsiveness to GH and cortisol. The severity of disordered pituitary function ran *pari passu* with the thyroid abnormalities, which ranged from just increased TSH levels to gross myxoedema.

An animal study has demonstrated that ovulation could be induced in aged female rats by L-dopa implants in the medial preoptic area (Cooper et al., 1979). The conclusion was that age-dependent disturbances of ovarian function could be initiated by changes in CNS neurotransmitters.

Baruch et al. (1976) have commented that digoxin may raise free-thyroxine-index (FTI) levels although this may involve direct cardiac effects rather than any TRH–TSH pathology. However, digoxin has a steroid-like structure and can cause gynaecomastia in men. Burckhardt et al. (1968) reported that digoxin can act on the pituitary, modifying gonadotrophin secretion. Although digoxin is now used more selectively than in the past it is still widely prescribed and it may have some as yet unrecognized effects on pituitary function.

Pituitary growth dynamic hormone (GDH) metabolism may be affected in chronic liver failure, but there is no evidence of any research on this topic in elderly subjects with liver disease (Baker et al., 1972).

The abnormal results of dynamic function tests of hypophyseal adreno-corticotrophic hormone (ACTH) secretory response in a younger subject taking indomethacin support the idea that prostaglandin precursors play a part in the hypothalamic control of ACTH (Beirne and Jubiz, 1978). Indomethacin is a cyclo-oxygenase inhibitor, affecting prostaglandin synthesis and thereby relieving pain, like so many of the analgesics used in geriatric as well as general medical practice.

Ramirez et al. (1976) have shown a defect in the hypophyseal response to TRH testing in chronic renal failure. They suggest this may be part of a more general pituitary effect rather than an isolated thyrotrophin abnormality. Hyperprolactinaemia has been described in chronic renal failure, more marked in the female subjects (Lim et al., 1979). The investigators thought that the abnormality was an abnormal stress response in the pituitary, which then became autonomous, but that there might also be a hypothalamic defect. Although uraemia is relatively common in old age, neither of these observations have been validated in the elderly.

All these findings suggest there may be many unsuspected 'cross-hormonal' abnormalities in the elderly due to multiple pathology and drug effects.

Pituitary-gonadal Function

Sociological and behavioural studies of sexual relationships outnumber the few studies of gonadal function in the elderly man and women. What evidence there is shows the follicle-stimulating hormone (FSH) levels rise in normally menstruating women many years before the menopause. FSH and luteinizing hormone (LH) levels then rise further post-menopausally, thus suggesting that the menopause is not as an abrupt event as was previously believed. High post-menopausal levels of FSH (130–660 mg LER–907/dl) and LH (15–60 mg LER–907/dl) are a normal anterior pituitary response to the failed target organ (Faiman et al., 1976); the menopause is an ovarian and not a pituitary problem. The high GDH levels may drop somewhat in extreme old age but are often sustained to the end of life, and we have found high levels in women of over 100.

There is only one large-scale study of the pituitary-gonadal function in elderly men (Baker et al., 1976). The findings suggested a primary decrease in testicular function over the age of 40, with testosterone levels falling showly in old age. Sex hormone binding globulin rose in old age, i.e. there was certainly no evidence of age-related carrier protein deficiency. In so far as the complicated issue of osteoporosis and sex hormones is concerned the testosterone–oestradiol conversion rate was increased rather than decreased. The substantial and long-maintained increment in gonadotrophin secretion is similar to that in older women.

There is no evidence that pituitary dysfunction is a common or re-mediable cause of the menopause or testicular failure, or of para-menopausal or climacteric problems, or of osteoporosis or arterial vascular disease sometimes ascribed to sex hormone lack. There is also no evidence that pituitary disease is linked to benign hypertrophy or carcinoma of the prostate, or to neoplasms of the breast, uterus or vagina. It is possible that gynaecomastia and even abnormal lactation might be associated with pituitary-gonadal, or pituitary-secondary sexual organ abnormalities in older people, but this has not been recorded.

A clinical feature of anorexia nervosa is amenorrhoea but with minimal or no gonadotrophin secretion. There is, as yet, no evidence that a similar condition occurs or would matter in malnutrition, anorectic or cachectic states in the elderly.

Posterior Pituitary

There is no reported evidence of disease of functional abnormality affecting oxytocin production in the elderly, nor of any hormonal deficiency caused by lack of the hypothalamic posterior pituitary hormone carrier proteins, the neurophysins. This includes reported cases of anterior pituitary dysfunction in older subjects.

Diabetes insipidus is a rare disease commonest in children, with only 10 per cent occurring after the age of 50 (Soffer, 1951). Tumours, usually secondary, are the most frequent cause of posterior pituitary antidiuretic hormone (ADH — vasopressin) lack in the older subject. The most common primaries are breast and bronchus (McKeown, 1965). However, abnormalities of ADH secretion, in the so-called syndrome of inappropriate ADH secretion — SIADH (which means the normal physiological controls of vasopressin secretion are disturbed) and of plasma volume, concentration, osmolarity and sodium levels, which may be caused by factors affecting the hypothalamic pituitary secretion of ADH and the peripheral renal action of the hormone, are common (*Fig.* 14.2*b*).

The diagnostic features of pituitary diabetes insipidus and the contrasting features of nephrogenic diabetes insipidus are summarized in *Table* 14.1. Both may occur in old age, sometimes both in the same elderly patient, and are probably often not recognized.

Hyponatraemia often used to be called asymptomatic before the SIADH concept was developed. It may not cause any obvious symptoms and may disappear if and when any concomitant illness is treated. However, hyponatraemia and low extracellular and total body sodium may be a cause of symptoms in their own right and may have widespread metabolic effects, since sodium is a major ionic component of plasma and extracellular fluid and is the main electrolyte factor in determining plasma osmolarity. The clinical effects of hyponatraemia are confusion, drowsiness, ataxia and dysphagia. The blood pressure may be raised and fits and coma may develop.

A high serum sodium is a rare finding in the elderly and is usually due to dehydration and hyperosmolar diabetic states. A low sodium is surprisingly common (Hodkinson, 1977) and although hypokalaemia has tended to attract more attention hyponatraemia should not be ignored, especially in ill old people. When hypokalaemia is present as well as hyponatraemia the low potassium could also be the result of SIADH. Mukherjee et al. (1973) have also found low sodium ion concentrations and defective osmoregulation in well elderly people. It is not appropriate here to discuss at length when, or how often, to carry out screening blood tests in old people. However, SIADH is one of several causes of potentially serious symptoms in older patients which can only be confirmed by blood tests and may not be suspected from the history and examination. The problem of abnormal homeostasis, discovered by blood tests, may be still very difficult to resolve as water retention and dilutional hyponatraemia (including fluid overload effects but also implying possible cranial or nephrogenic ADH abnormalities) may be present in the same patient. For instance, cardiac failure may lead to lowered renal blood flow but renal impairment and the use of diuretics and other drugs that may affect the pituitary and/or kidney may produce a complicated picture.

In SIADH the low sodium is associated with high urinary osmolarity

Table 14.1. Features of diabetes insipidus

	Cranial	*Nephrogenic*

Causes	Tumour
	1° Pituitary
	  Craniopharyngioma
	
	2° Breast
	  Bronchus
	Infection
	  TB
	  Syphilis
	  Encephalitis
	'Inflammatory'
	  Sarcoid
	Trauma
	  Head injury
		Hyperkalaemia
		Hypokalaemia
		Chronic renal failure
		Obstructive uropathy
		Prolonged overhydration
		Lithium

Features	Polydipsia, Polyuria normal or high plasma osmolarity	
	Little change in urine osmolarity, serum osmolarity rises, with water deprivation	No change in urine osmolarity with water deprivation
	Normal water load excretion after vasopressin	Unable to excrete water load after vasopressin
	Urine osmolarity rises after vasopressin, not necessarily to normal	No change in urine osmolarity after vasopressin
	Beware. Do not do water deprivation tests in severely dehydrated patients	
Treatment	1. Substitution with modified ADH/vasopressin: DDAVP (desmopressin) has minimal vasoconstrictor effect. Given intranasally or intramuscularly 2. Chlorpropamide (and other drugs potentiating ADH – *see Fig.* 12.2*b*) but may produce hypoglycaemia	Thiazides – only treatment available. Watch for potassium depletion

and loss of sodium in the urine, and is not helped by supplementary sodium. Inappropriate excessive posterior-pituitary ADH secretion is usually the cause, but renal sensitivity to normal ADH levels may be a factor, and ectopic ADH secretion can also occur. In the latter other carcinomatous effects of neoplastic illness and abnormal ACTH production could produce confusing symptoms and signs and could also effect the sodium levels.

Minor and serious examples of SIADH are common in old people. The main causes of SIADH in the elderly are shown in *Table* 14.2. The important message is that the hyponatraemia can cause symptoms and is more common than most doctors realize.

SIADH/dilutional hyponatraemia is characterized by the urinary osmolarity exceeding that of the plasma with a sustained high urinary sodium excretion. This must be distinguished from salt-deficient states. In the latter the patient is dehydrated, the blood urea is usually raised and

Table 14.2. Causes of SIADH

Excessive ADH Secretion

    Chest infections
    Congestive cardiac failure
    Hypothyroidism
    Cerebral   trauma
              neoplasm
              infections
    CVAs?
    Psychotic states

Drugs (excessive ADH secretion or altered renal sensitivity)

    Chlorpropamide
    Tricyclic antidepressants
    Thiazides
    Carbamazepine
    Clofibrate

Ectopic ADH

    Carcinoma bronchus
               pancreas
               duodenum
               ureter
    Pulmonary tuberculosis

there may be postural hypotension. However, as already described, CCF and thiazides may produce SIADH. Patients with chronic debilitating diseases may have a varient of SIADH as a result of actual downward resetting of 'the osmostat' (DeFronzo et al., 1976). The osmoreceptors controlling ADH secretion appeared to act at a lower level of serum osmolarity in this study; the resulting hyponatraemia was reported as asymptomatic.

The treatment of SIADH is obviously to try and remove any primary conditions, but symptomatic treatment to restore plasma osmolarity is usually required. This is by fluid retention, sometimes to less than 500 ml daily, by the use of sodium-retaining steroids such as alpha-fludrocortisone in largish doses of the order of 0·5—1 mg/d, and sometimes supplementary salt, which is best given as slow release sodium in an attempt to minimize any nausea and vomiting.

HYPOTHERMIA

Impaired response to cold stress or frank hypothermia could be the presenting feature of hypopituitarism and primary or secondary hypothyroidism, but these have been thought to be rare causes of reduced cold-stress response and hypothermia in old age. Emslie-Smith and McClean (1977), in reviewing the disorders predisposing to hypothermia, mention that a variety of intracranial lesions may interfere with temperature homeostasis. These include strokes, subdural haematomas, cerebral neoplasms, cerebral trauma and Parkinson's disease. Hypothermia is most likely in lesions involving the third ventricle (Matthews, 1967), or the hypothalamus itself (Keoppen et al., 1969).

Wernicke's encephalopathy may involve the hypothalamus. Excessive alcohol consumption does occur in the elderly and could lead to hypothermia in those at risk by causing peripheral vasodilatation, confusion and carelessness, and immobilizing falls even without a central lesion. Chronic brain failure (dementia) could have centrally acting effects contributing to hypothermia as well as causing carelessness leading to self neglect and a risk of hypothermia.

Many drugs have been blamed for hypothermia; these include chlorpromazine, tricyclic antidepressants and benzodiazepines. These drugs probably act centrally affecting vasoconstrictor responses, but they can affect hypothalamic function, e.g. by causing hyperprolactinaemia.

Fox (1974) has reviewed the present understanding of temperature regulation in man. Animal research has suggested that monoamines in the hypothalamus are important in temperature regulation, both in controlling hypothalamic activity and as hypothalamic messengers to other parts of the body. These include 5HT, noradrenaline and prostaglandins, and they probably act on, or are transmitted by, an anterior hypothalamic thermostat. Work by Feldberg et al. (1970) has shown that a temperature set-point is probably located in the posterior hypothalamus and that sodium and calcium ions, and particularly their ratio in the extracellular fluid, are the most important controlling factors. Influences from the mid-brain, peripheral heat production and loss, and the effects of drugs, pyrogens and above all the blood temperature, are other important influences on the hypothalamus. Hypothermia and cold intolerance have been induced in animals by a hypothalamic peptide, neurotensin, which may act directly on the CNS or affect peripheral vasculature (Bissette et al., 1976).

Unfortunately, once again it has to be said that there is as yet no definite link between these research observations and their endocrine and clinical significance in older people.

AGEING

It is generally taught that people only become endocrinologically ill, and even die, in old age if they truly have hyper- or hypoglandular states. However, it has long been believed that glandular extracts might reverse, slow down or prevent ageing in a more non-specific way acting on the body generally, or on organs such as the gonads. Many proponents of this supposition have wondered whether thyroid extract might be an anti-ageing elixir, and have been supported by the finding of atrophic changes in the gland. The thyroid reacts normally to TSH in the elderly but it is now suggested that a pituitary defect in TSH production might be a senescent change; there is no confirmatory evidence of this.

Just to confuse the issue, hypophysectomy actually retards the ageing of collagen (Everitt and Olsen, 1965). Animal experiments suggest that ageing still continues in hypophysectomized rats, but is retarded (Verzar and Spichtin, 1966). These results may not have been due to any direct pituitary hormonal effect as hypophysectomized animals eat less and this may have been the cause of the retarded ageing.

REFERENCES

Andrew W. (1971) *The Anatomy of Ageing in Man and Animals.* New York and London, Heinemann.
Baker H. W. G., Burger H. G., DeKretser D. M. et al. (1976) *Clin. Endocrinol.* 5, 349.
Baker H. W. G., Dulmanis A., Hudson B. et al. (1972) *Abstracts of Fourth International Congress of Endocrinology, No. 327,* Amsterdam, Excerpta Medica.
Baruch A. L. H., Davis C. and Hodkinson H. M. (1976) *Age Ageing* 5, 224.
Beirne J. and Jubiz W. (1978) *Clin. Endocrinol. Metabol.* 47, 713.
Berthaux P., Beck H., Levillain R. et al. (1962) *Sem. Hôp. Paris,* 38, 1410.
Bigos S. T., Ridgway C., Kourides I. A. et al. (1977) *Clin. Endocrinol. Metabol.* 46, 317.
Bissette G., Nemeroff C. B., Loosen P. T. et al. (1976) *Nature* 262, 607.
Burckhardt D., Vera C. A. and Ladue J. S. (1968) *Ann. Intern. Med.* 68, 1069.
Calderon L., Ryan N. and Kovacs K. (1978) *Gerontology* 24, 441.
Coni N. K. (1973) *Mod. Geriatr.* 3, 544.
Cooper R. L., Brandt F. J., Linnoila M. et al. (1979) *Neuroendocrinology* 28, 234.
Costello R. T. (1936) *Am. J. Pathol.* 12, 205.
DeFronzo R. A., Goldberg M. and Angus Z. S. (1976) *Ann. Intern. Med.* 84, 538.
Eddy R. L., Jones A. L., Chakmakjian Z. N. et al. (1974) *J. Clin. Endocrinol.* 33, 709.
Everitt A. V. and Olsen G. G. (1965) *Nature* 206, 307.
Emslie Smith D. and MacLean D. (1977) *Accidental Hypothermia.* Philadelphia, Lippincott.
Exton-Smith A. N. (1972) Personal communication.
Faiman C., Winter J. D. and Reyes F. I. (1976) In: Baird D. T. (ed.), *Clinics in Obstetrics and Gynaecology* 3(3), Philadelphia, Saunders.
Feldberg W., Myers R. D. and Veale W. L. (1970) *J. Physiol.* 207, 403.
Fox R. H. (1974) In: R. J. Linden (ed.), *Recent Advances in Physiology.* Edinburgh and London, Churchill Livingstone.
Hodkinson H. M. (1974) *Gerontol. Clin. (Basel)* 16, 175.
Hodkinson H. M. (1977) *Biochemical Diagnosis of the Elderly.* London, Chapman & Hall.

Hsu K. H. and Peng M. T. (1978) *Gerontology* **24**, 434.
Keoppen A. H., Tentler R. L., Barron K. D. et al. (1969) *Postgrad. Med.* **46**, 183.
Kernohan J. W. and Sayre G. P. (1956) *Tumours of the Pituitary Gland and Infundibulum.* Armed Forces Institute of Pathology.
Laron Z., Doron M. and Amikan B. (1970) *Medicine and Sport, 4.* Basel, Petah Tigra-Karger, pp. 126–131.
Lim V. S., Kathpalia S. C. and Frohman L. A. (1979) *J. Clin. Endocrinol. Metabol.* **48**, 101.
McKeown F. (1965) *Pathology of the Aged.* London, Butterworths.
Maisey I. and Stevens A. (1969) *Guy's Hosp. Rep.* **118**, 373.
Matthews J. A. (1967) *Postgrad Med. J.* **43**, 662.
Mukherjee A. P., Coni N. K. and Davison W. (1973) *Gerontol. Clin. (Basel)* **15**, 227.
Ngu J. L. and Paley R. G. (1968) *Geriatrics* **23**, 166.
Ramirez G., O'Neill W. jun., Jubiz W. et al. (1976) *Ann. Intern. Med.* **84**, 672.
Soffer L. J. (1951) *Diseases of the Endocrine Glands.* London, Kimpton.
Soffer L. J., Dorfman R. I. and Gabrilove J. L. (1961) *The Human Adrenal Gland.* London, Kimpton.
Verzar F. and Spichtin H. (1966) *Gerontologia* **12**, 48.
Zerney C. J. (1957) *Canad. Med. Assoc. J.* **76**, 962.

15. ADRENAL FUNCTION AND DISEASES
M. F. Green

The pituitary—adrenal axis has already been described in Chapter 14 (*see Fig.* 14.1). This axis is particularly important in the body's reaction to stressful stimuli. It is often alleged that there is a decline in the response of aged individuals to a variety of stresses, and even that hypoadrenalism may be a cause of senescence. Certainly, some of the 'normal' stress reactions may not occur in ill old people, e.g. raised white count, tachycardia and fever in those with infections. Signs suggestive of adrenal lack such as marked skin pigmentation, hypotension, confusion and loss of body hair are all common findings in the elderly. Addisonian hypoadrenalism can occur either in its own right or after treatment for Cushing's disease in older patients.

There is, however, no evidence that these clinical features, modified stress responses, or the premature ageing states of progeria and Werner's syndrome are due to impaired pituitary or adrenocortical function. Indeed, our own research has shown that ill old people seem to have normally raised cortisol levels compatible with effective pituitary adrenal response. Nevertheless, certain illnesses occurring in the elderly may be associated with impaired hypophyso-adrenal response including malnutrition and depression.

Corticosteroid treatment may, of course, be indicated, e.g. in shocked patients (but *see* hypothermia, p. 197) and in elderly people suffering from conditions such as rheumatoid arthritis and pemphigus. The doses used are normally non-physiological and are not particularly intended to correct any adrenal insufficiency. There has been a vogue for using the sodium-retaining mineralocorticoid alphafludrocortisone in the treatment of postural hypotension not caused by drugs and sometimes alleged to be due to total body sodium depletion. There is no evidence that this condition is caused by adrenal disease. It is more likely to be due to an age-related failure of baroreceptors; 'getting-up slowly', heavy-duty waist length tights and even salt supplements may be more useful.

HISTOPATHOLOGY AND HISTOPHYSIOLOGY
A review by Hall (1978) and the findings of Dobbie (1969) suggest that adrenocortical nodularity is much commoner than suggested by McKeown (1965), who only described four abnormal adrenals in her series. Dobbie

described nodules, sometimes multiple, and sometimes as large as 20 mm diameter, present in 14 per cent of consecutive post mortems in the elderly, with 80 per cent of the 50—80-year-olds showing capsular artery obliteration. Hypertensive damage seemed to be the usual cause. The histological features of the nodules were degenerative and likely to be associated with deficient hormone production, although adrenal cortical adenomata can be secretory and could produce Cushing's disease. This has rarely been described in old age.

Hypoadrenalism in older people may be associated with long-term survival of patients treated when younger. In newly discovered aged victims autoimmune disease may be the cause. There is a well known association between autoimmune disease and raised autoantibodies to other organs, sometimes resulting in actual disease.

The adrenal cortex contains high levels of vitamin C and it has been suggested that ascorbic acid is required for steroid synthesis. Many old people, in and out of hospital, have lowered leucocyte ascorbic acid (LAA) levels and/or symptoms ascribable to possible vitamin C lack. Dubin et al. (1978) found no evidence of adrenocortical insufficiency in elderly patients with low LAA levels, as judged by tetracosactrin (Synacthen) stimulation tests, and there was no change in the results after vitamin C supplements.

PITUITARY—ADRENAL FUNCTION TESTS

The functions and relationships of the cerebro—hypothalamic—pituitary—adrenocortical axis and the common tests used in assessing the competence of the axis are shown in *Fig.* 15.1. Important stresses in elderly people are cold, malnutrition, surgery and acute and chronic illnesses including infections, strokes and depression.

In view of the dynamic nature of the pituitary—adrenal relationship and the variation of adrenocorticotrophic hormone (ACTH) levels with the interplay of the likely stresses, it is customary to rely on tests which measure several values of cortisol during stimulation or suppression of hypothalamic—pituitary or adrenal function. There do appear to be some age-related abnormalities in studies in animals and humans, particularly affecting the functional reserve capacity of the pituitary—adrenal axis or the response to one only of several tests.

Animal experiments have suggested that resting corticosteroid levels are normally maintained in aged rats and dogs (Hess and Riegle, 1970; Bresnock and McQueen, 1970). However, the response to stimulation tests suggests an age-related decline in adrenocortical response.

A few human studies of pituitary and adrenocortical responsiveness in well old people have not shown any such impairment of functional reserve capacity. Friedman et al. (1969) investigated fit ambulant convalescent patients measuring plasma cortisol levels in the resting state, after stimulation with insulin-induced hypoglycaemia, ACTH and tetracosactrin, and after dexamethasone suppression. There was no evidence of any pituitary

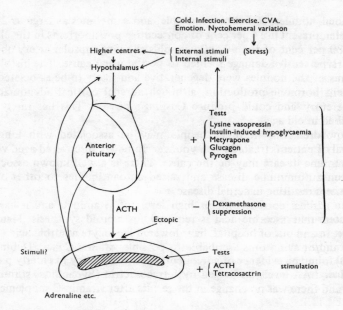

Fig. 15.1. Pituitary–adrenal relationships.

or adrenal deficiency or unresponsiveness. The only abnormality was a higher sleeping midnight cortisol level than in younger subject. Blichert-Toft (1975) and Blichert-Toft and Hummer (1977) have confirmed earlier findings that the intravenous (IV) metyrapone test is a useful and safe way of investigating pituitary–adrenal function in old age.

Blichert-Toft (1975) has surveyed his own previous work and that of other researchers, looking particularly at elderly patients undergoing surgery, and similarly found no evidence of adrenal insufficiency or need for pituitary–adrenal supplementation. He did not find any noticeable decline in circulating ACTH in older subjects.

Hall (1978) has reviewed published measurements of cortisol utilization and clearance in the aged which suggest that there may be an age-related defect in adrenal responsiveness to stimulation and in the elimination of circulating cortisone. This may have been due to reduced basal metabolism or liver cortisol clearance, or to decreased muscle bulk implying lessened cortisol utilization.

None of the published research findings suggests any constant and treatable effects affecting the hypophyso-adreno-cortical axis.

ADRENAL GLAND AND MALIGNANT DISEASE

The ectopic production of ACTH most commonly occurs in association with carcinoma of the bronchus (especially oat cell), a neoplasm relatively common in old age. Ectopic ACTH secretion has also been found with breast, gastrointestinal and urogenital neoplasms. Three subjects of the ten with bronchogenic carcinoma associated with abnormal ACTH secretion, studied by Singer et al. (1978) were aged 65 or more. These ten had been identified from 164 patients with bronchogenic carcinoma. The ectopic hormone condition is often not recognized because Cushingoid features rarely develop or the neoplasm itself produces other disabling symptoms.

The clinical features are due to the excessive and often rapidly rising levels of ACTH causing a hypochloraemic hypokalaemic alkalosis, with thirst and polyuria, cachexia, myopathy, tachycardia and oedema (this oedema is presumably due to the glucocorticoid-induced sodium retention, but also possibly caused by the hypoalbuminaemia of severe illness). The majority of the subjects were also hyperglycaemic. Many died within 7–12 days.

It is important to remember the possibility of the diagnosis in ill old people with characteristically disordered electrolytes, especially if lung cancer is thought to be present. The abnormal ACTH levels which can be assayed, and are usually much higher than in Cushing's disease, are sustained throughout the 24 hours and are not suppressible. It may be possible to help the symptoms caused by the excessive ACTH by aminoglutethimide and sometimes with metyrapone; spironolactone may reduce symptoms associated with hypokalaemia.

ADRENAL MEDULLA

There have only been two reports of phaeochromocytoma occurring in old age (Eisenberg and Wallerstein, 1932; McKeown, 1965), and no instances of any other adrenal medullary disorder. Fisher (1971) investigated urinary vanillyl-mandelic acid (VMA) excretion in elderly subjects and found little change with advancing age, suggesting good preservation of normal adrenal medullary secretion.

HYPOTHERMIA

There is no evidence that hypoadrenalism plays an important part in the aetiology of hypothermia. However, corticosteroids, usually given as large doses of hydrocortisone, have been used as a supportive measure in shocked hypothermic patients – and hypothermia is a serious and often lethal disease. Corticosteroids have similarly been used in the treatment of other serious conditions which may occur in the elderly, such as Gram-negative septicaemias. There is no good evidence as to their efficacy in these situations.

Mills (1976) tried to include the use of corticosteroids in a controlled trial of treating hypothermia during a long-term study of patients admitted to the Central Middlesex Hospital. The initial evidence, of no statistical significance, suggested that corticosteroids might be harmful and the attempt was abandoned.

REFERENCES

Blichert-Toft M. (1975) *Acta Endocrinol.* [suppl.] (Kbh.) 195.
Blichert-Toft M. and Hummer L. (1977) *Gerontology* 23, 236.
Bresnock E. M. and McQueen R. D. (1970) *Am. J. Vet. Res.* 31, 1269.
Dobbie J. W. (1969) *J. Pathol. Bact.* 99, 1.
Dubin W. J., MacLennan W. J. and Hamilton J. C. (1978) *Gerontology* 24, 473.
Eisenberg A. A. and Wallerstein H. (1932) *Arch. Pathol.* 14, 818.
Fisher R. H. (1971) *Gerontol. Clin.* (*Basel*) 13, 257.
Friedman M., Green M. F. and Sharland E. (1969) *J. Gerontol.* 24, 292.
Hall M. R. P. (1978) In: Brocklehurst J. C. (ed.), *Textbook of Geriatric Medicine and Gerontology.* 2nd ed. Edinburgh and London, Churchill Livingstone, p. 456.
Hess G. D. and Riegle G. B. (1970) *J. Gerontol.* 25, 354.
McKeown F. (1965) *Pathology of the Aged.* London, Butterworths.
Mills G. (1976) Personal communication.
Singer W., Kovacs K., Ryan N. et al. (1978) *J. Clin. Pathol.* 31, 591.

16. THYROID FUNCTION
J. A. Thomson

OUTLINE OF CURRENT VIEWS OF THYROID PHYSIOLOGY
The Thyroid Gland

Although several other tissues in the body such as the gastric mucosa, the salivary gland and the lactating breast can all trap iodide, the thyroid gland in the human is the only organ capable of the complete synthesis of the thyroid hormones thyroxine (tetraiodothyronine, T_4) and triiodothyronine (T_3). The thyroid is mainly under the control of the pituitary which produces the hormone thyrotrophin (thyroid-stimulating hormone, TSH). This stimulates both the growth of the thyroid cells and also several stages in the formation of the thyroid hormones. These hormones have in turn a negative feedback effect on the pituitary so that the administration of either T_4 or T_3 in sufficient dosage will suppress the release of TSH from the pituitary. In turn the pituitary is influenced from the hypothalamus by means of the hypothalamic-releasing hormone, thyrotrophin-releasing hormone (TRH) which stimulates the release of TSH from the pituitary. The hypothalamus is controlled by a negative feedback response from the thyroid hormones and also is influenced by higher centres, but the controlling mechanisms have not yet been defined.

The thyroid gland is not entirely under higher control. It has a certain amount of autonomous function. For instance, it can be shown in the experimental animal that in the absence of the pituitary the thyroid is capable of responding to iodine deficiency by showing increasing trapping of iodine and contrastingly when exposed to sudden large doses of iodine the gland is capable of shutting off hormone synthesis by stopping organic binding of iodine in the thyroid (Wolff–Chaikoff effect). These two mechanisms clearly are of importance in attempting to maintain an equilibrium in the level of thyroid hormones in the face of the widely varying iodine contents of the diet.

The mechanisms of hormone synthesis within the thyroid have been reviewed on many occasions. A recent comprehensive review is that by De Groot and Niepomniszcze (1977). The steps in the biosynthesis pathway are:

1. The trapping of iodide.
2. The transformation of iodide into an active form. This seems to be dependent on a peroxidase enzyme system.

3. The incorporation of this iodine into thyroxine to give mono- and diiodotyrosine (MIT and DIT).

4. The coupling of MIT and DIT to form T_3 and T_4 as part of the thyroglobulin molecule.

5. The breakdown of thyroglobulin, as required, by a protease enzyme system to release T_4 and T_3 into the plasma.

6. The conservation of iodine by the breakdown of MIT and DIT by the dehalogenase enzyme system.

Our knowledge of the above steps of thyroid hormone biosynthesis has been largely derived from the use of radioactive isotopes of iodide for kinetic studies, especially in patients with inherited enzymatic defects of thyroid hormone biosynthesis (Stanbury and Talley, 1977). The other useful tools have been drugs with specific actions on the thyroid, such as potassium perchlorate and thiocyanate which block the accumulation of iodide from the plasma and also discharge from the gland any non-organified iodide, and drugs of the thiocarbamide series which block the iodination of tyrosine but do not interfere with trapping of iodide from the blood.

The Peripheral Metabolism of Thyroid Hormones

When T_3 and T_4 are released into the circulation they travel bound to proteins of the plasma. This binding system has been reviewed by Robbins (1975). The main binding protein is thyroxine binding globulin (TBG). This is the protein which has the highest specificity of binding although it has a limited binding capacity. The other major binding protein is thyroxine binding pre-albumin (TBPA) which has a lower specificity of binding but a higher binding capacity than TBG. It also seems to be more susceptible to change in acute situations such as during operations or severe illnesses when usually TBG does not alter significantly. The other binding protein of note is albumin, which has a large binding capacity for thyroxine but a very low specificity of binding. It is not clear whether albumin binding plays any significant role in thyroid homeostasis.

The importance of these binding proteins is that well over 99 per cent of the T_4 and T_3 in peripheral blood is carried in a protein bound form. The bound fraction is considered to be in equilibrium with a very small free hormone fraction and it would seem likely that the free hormone is the active component determining the metabolic effect, although final proof of this hypothesis is not yet available. Because T_3 is bound to a lesser extent than T_4 to the plasma proteins the proportion of unbound T_3 is significantly higher than T_4.

The secretion of the thyroid gland is unusual in that two hormones, T_4 and T_3, with a similar metabolic effect are produced. It is, therefore, important to examine the evidence for the relationship between these two substances. If one examines the constituents in the thyroid gland T_4 is present in excess of T_3. Similarly, in the peripheral blood T_4 is present in higher concentration than T_3. Experiments have shown that when either T_4 or T_3 is given to a hypothyroid animal there is a delay before there is a metabolic response, and that this delay is greater when T_4 is given. Some authors take the view that the role of T_4 is merely as a pro-hormone for T_3. Thus the current view is that although the main secretion of the thyroid gland is T_4 with a small amount of T_3, in the periphery, most, if not all, thyroxine is transformed to T_3.

T_3 is thought to exert the feedback control on the pituitary and hypothalamus. Other authors have, however, argued that there is evidence that in some states the important factor controlling the metabolic response is T_4 and not T_3. For instance, where there is a failing thyroid such as after ^{131}I treatment, thyroidectomy or with thyroiditis, the T_4 falls; the T_3 is often elevated to try and compensate and the TSH is also elevated. In this situation if the T_3 had been the important feedback factor one would have anticipated a raised T_3 suppressing TSH production from the pituitary, but in this instance TSH release seems to have been stimulated by the low level of thyroxine.

One further complication has been from the development of assays for reverse T_3 $(3, 3', 5' T_3)$. This substance in contrast to T_3 $(3, 5, 3' T_3)$ has one iodinated site on the inner ring and two iodinated sites on the outer ring. All the available evidence would point to this substance being virtually inert metabolically. It appears that it is formed from the breakdown of T_4 and thus gives a fine peripheral control of metabolic effect whereby T_4 alternatively could be metabolized to the highly active T_3 or the virtually inactive reverse T_3.

The peripheral effect of thyroid hormones has not been well defined. The hormones have effects on a variety of metabolic processes, but no primary action has been found. Attempts have been made to study the binding of T_4 and T_3 by various tissues. Separate binding proteins seem to exist for both substances and there is some evidence that, in areas such as the hypothalamus, T_3 has preferential access to the cells and especially to the cell nuclei. Therefore, in theory it would be in a better position to influence cellular metabolism than T_4, which is not so bound. In contrast, in other tissues there are specific cytosol binding proteins for T_4; and so perhaps there is variation in which of the two hormones is important in any particular organ.

TESTS OF THYROID FUNCTION
Serum Thyroxine
Since quantitatively thyroxine is the major thyroid hormone techniques for its estimation have been available for some years. Originally this was done indirectly by means of the protein bound iodine (PBI) which allowed an estimation of the thyroxine present in a serum sample by means of estimation of its iodine content. Because of the various substances interfering with the PBI estimation (Davis, 1966) and because of the development

of more specific methods of measuring serum thyroxine, the PBI estimation is now virtually of historical interest.

The serum thyroxine is usually now estimated by means of a radioimmunoassay technique, although competitive binding methods are still widely used. Normal values are of the order of 55—144 nmol/l.

Serum Triiodothyronine
This is usually estimated by a radioimmunoassay technique. The serum total T_3 level is of the order of 0·8—2·8 nmol/l.

Reverse T_3
At certain centres radioimmunoassays for this substance have been developed. The normal range is 0·15—0·42 nmol/l in Glasgow Royal Infirmary (Ratcliffe et al., 1976) but there is no general agreement between different centres about normal ranges.

Free Thyroid Hormone Estimations
If one accepts that there is a free portion of both T_4 and T_3 and that these are the fractions which control the metabolic effect, it would be advantageous to be able to measure these directly. Techniques to do this have been developed, but most of them are cumbersome, rendering them unsuitable for routine use, although simplified kits are now coming into use.

T_3 Resin Tests
The value of these tests are that they allow estimation of the unsaturated part of thyroxine binding proteins to be made. This is important in various states when the binding protein is altered, the most important of these being on the pill or during pregnancy in which the TBG concentration is increased due to oestrogens; or, in contrast, in the nephrotic syndrome; or following the administration of androgens, when the TBG level is decreased. In these conditions falsely high or falsely low serum T_4 and T_3 values respectively would be found. The combination of a serum thyroxine estimation and a T_3 resin test allows one to compensate for the alteration in the binding proteins and in effect obtain a corrected thyroxine value.

TSH Estimations
Since the TSH output from the pituitary provides a sensitive reflection of the pituitary response to low levels of thyroid hormone it is not surprising that radioimmunoassay techniques of TSH estimation have gained in popularity in the estimation of minor degrees of thyroid failure. There is some variability between laboratories, but values of the order of 0—8 mu/l have been found. It should be noted that estimation is of no value in the diagnosis of thyrotoxicosis since the sensitivity at the lower end of the assay is not such that a clear discrimination between the low-normal levels and frankly suppressed levels can be made.

TRH Tests

The administration of synthetic tripeptide TRH has gained in popularity in recent years as a test of thyroid function especially in the diagnosis of minor degrees of thyrotoxicosis. The test is performed following the intravenous injection of the drug and the response of the patient's serum TSH is monitored over the next 60 minutes. In the normal individual there is a brisk response in the serum TSH value reaching a peak at 20 min and returning towards normal at 1 hour. In the presence of thyroid failure there is an elevated basal level of TSH coupled with an excessive response to the TRH stimulus. Conversely in thyrotoxicosis the high levels of thyroid hormones have suppressed both the pituitary and the hypothalamus, thus resulting in a low basal value of TSH and an absent response to the stimulus. Sometimes in hypothalamic disease a result giving a delayed response with a maximal level of TSH being found at 60 rather than 20 min is found.

Thus the TRH test has been looked upon as a test of the overall metabolic effect of the thyroid hormones using the hypothalamus as a target tissue.

Radioiodine Studies

In the 1950s radioiodine studies were the main form of thyroid function tests. With the advent of precise biochemical measurements these have fallen largely into disuse as a routine, although in patients who are to have therapeutic radioactive iodine the uptake of the tracer dose is one of the factors used in calculating a therapeutic dose of radioiodine.

The normal range of radioiodine uptake was usually quoted at around 15–45 per cent of the administered dose at 24 hours. There is evidence, however, that with increasing iodine consumption in various forms that the average uptake has fallen significantly over the last two decades. Apart from the 24 h uptake other uptake times were used, particularly early uptake times, such as 20 min to 4 h in the diagnosis of thyrotoxicosis and 48 h in the diagnosis of hypothyroidism.

Studies using radioactive isotopes can also be supplemented by various stimulatory tests, such as a TSH stimulation test which was used to see whether one could increase the uptake of radioactive iodine by the injection of bovine TSH. The implication was that if the uptake could be increased it would be unlikely that the patient was suffering from primary thyroid failure. This test has been almost entirely superseded by estimation of the serum TSH.

Conversely, the various types of suppression test where one administered exogenous thyroid hormone, particularly T_3, and measured the thyroid uptake before and following a 10-day course of the hormone were widely used in the diagnosis of autonomous thyroid function. Characteristically in thyrotoxicosis non-suppressibility of the uptake was found. This test has been largely replaced by the TRH test, although detailed studies have shown that the tests do not measure identical aspects of thyroid control.

Formerly radioiodine studies included not only an estimation of thyroid uptake but also an estimation of the serum protein bound ^{131}I at 48 h. This gave a crude index of the rate of turnover of iodine within the thyroid, an accelerated turnover being found in thyrotoxicosis and in situations where the reserve of thyroid tissue was diminished, such as in Hashimoto's thyroiditis or following surgery or radioiodine treatment or alternatively in the presence of a single autonomous thyroid nodule. This test, however, has largely fallen into disuse.

Thyroid Scanning

Thyroid scanning is now the major situation in which one would use in vivo radioisotope studies. The clinical indications for such studies are the presence of a solitary thyroid nodule or a difference in consistency between different parts of the thyroid gland or following removal of a differentiated thyroid cancer to delineate any thyroid tissue remaining after operation.

Formerly ^{131}I was the main isotope used for scanning as it was also used for thyroid uptake and turnover studies. Now technetium (^{99m}Tc) is the main isotope used for scanning because the physical characteristics of its gamma emission is more suitable for good quality thyroid scans. Since, however, technetium is handled differently in the thyroid than iodine the two uptake patterns may not be exactly comparable. Iodine, in the normal thyroid, is rapidly organically bound whereas technetium is not protein bound to any significant extent. Therefore on some occasions differences between the technetium scan and the ^{131}I scan have been found, where the ^{131}I scan gave a 'hot' scan and the technetium scan gave a result implying a non-functional lesion because of the particular time it was done.

Tests for Thyroid Antibodies

Over the last 20 years a variety of techniques have been described for measuring thyroid antibodies. The original test involved the demonstration of a precipitating antibody to thyroglobulin by means of an agar gel technique. Subsequently tanned red cell agglutination tests and, more recently, radioimmunoassay tests for thyroglobulin antibodies have been developed. In addition complement fixing antibodies have been demonstrated against thyroid microsomes, as have antibodies against other portions of thyroid tissue, both in the colloid and in the cell. However, the most important tests in clinical practice are those directed against thyroglobulin and those directed against the thyroid microsomes. The problem with thyroid antibody tests is that although it is not uncommon to find low titre results the clinical significance of such a finding is not very high. On the other hand the finding of very strongly positive thyroid antibodies in a patient who has the clinical picture suggestive of autoimmunizing thyroiditis provides good confirmatory evidence for the diagnosis. One complicating feature is that thyroiditis does not exclude thyroid malignancy. The two have been found to coexist in a significant number of patients and, therefore, one has to take the whole clinical picture into account before reaching a definitive diagnosis.

FACTORS AFFECTING THYROID FUNCTION TESTS

In this section it is proposed to review current data on alteration of thyroid function tests in older subjects, excluding however the changes brought about by thyroid disease. These are dealt with in the succeeding chapter.

Problems of 'Normal' Ranges

One problem common to this field, as to all others which involve biochemical measurements is the question of how one chooses a normal range. Traditionally normal ranges were estimated by taking a population of healthy subjects apparently free from any disease and not on any medications. These subjects were often groups such as blood donors, medical students, technical, nursing and medical staff but, as will be obvious, these various groups of possibly normal people do not usually include subjects in the geriatric age group. It has been found in studies with autoanalysers that the majority of results which fell slightly outside the normal range were in the older patient and probably did not indicate the presence of disease. We have unfortunately only very limited data with respect to thyroid function tests.

Where an abnormal test is found in an older patient the question which has to be answered is whether this deviation from the normal range is explicable on the basis of age *per se* or whether it indicates disease. This is a difficult if not impossible question to answer because surveys of apparently healthy old people have shown a significant occurrence of various diseases of increasing incidence with age. In addition the older person is likely to be on a variety of medications for these diseases or indeed on a variety of self-administered medicines. If one, however, accepts these defects, there has accumulated certain information on the apparent effect of age on thyroid function tests.

With respect to thryroid gland function itself there is evidence that the radioiodine uptake falls with increasing age (Gaffney et al., 1962). These studies have been supplemented by more detailed work on the renal excretion, absolute iodine uptake and hormone degradation rates in older people (Gaffney et al., 1962; Hansen et al., 1975). These studies have shown that the thyroid radioiodide clearance and absolute iodine uptake fall with increasing age. There is a coincidental decrease in renal clearance of radioiodine which results in a relatively higher plasma inorganic iodine in older people. This tends relatively to preserve the radioiodine uptake. Metabolic equilibrium is maintained by a reduced T_4 degradation rate.

Levels of thyroid hormones in the peripheral blood as measured by protein bound iodine estimations (Tucker and Keys, 1951) showed that the PBI gradually decreased with increasing age. This was confirmed in more recent studies by Jeffereys et al. (1972) who showed that in almost 500 patients admitted to a geriatric department approximately one-fifth had subnormal PBI values. In most this seemed to be due to alteration of the TBG levels. It should be noted that this study was performed in patients admitted to a geriatric unit and, therefore, does introduce the complication of other illnesses affecting the results. In contrast, in studies performed from Glasgow (Thomson et al., 1972) of estimation of the PBI in apparently healthy people at home, the problem was not low PBI values but elevated levels. These seemed to be mainly due to problems with the normal range alluded to above and also to problems with administration of iodine-containing drugs such as cough medicines.

These studies in respect to the PBI have more recently been supplemented by estimations of the serum total thyroxine and T_3 levels. Overall it has been found that serum thyroxine levels do not fall significantly in healthy people with advancing age. Indeed recently it has been suggested (Burrows et al., 1975) that in older people there is a state of T_4 euthyroidism that is that the serum T_3 level is often low and that therefore the serum T_4 level is raised to compensate for this. This view has been challenged by other authors but has been confirmed on a population survey by Evered et al. (1978).

Studies of the free thyroid hormone concentrations (Herrmann et al., 1974) have shown slightly low serum free T_4 but significantly low both total and free serum T_3 values in elderly patients. Thus there would seem to be a trend for the serum T_3 to be much more affected by age than serum T_4. This view has been challenged by Olsen et al. (1978).

Limited studies have been done of the serum TSH and TRH responses in older people. The serum TSH increases with age (Ohara et al., 1974; Evered et al., 1978) but studies from the Newcastle group have shown that the rise in serum TSH is probably not dependent on age itself but is likely to reflect subclinical thyroiditis with marginal impairment in the thyroid function. Studies using TRH have shown that there can be both an excessive response of TSH to TRH administration (Ohara et al., 1974), probably indicating subclinical thyroid failure, or a diminished response (Snyder and Utiger, 1972).

Influence of Non Endocrine Disease

A problem that has been recognized for some years has been the presence of low circulating thyroid hormone levels in the 'sick' euthyroid subject, that is the patient who by all clinical criteria is euthyroid and who has some severe intercurrent illness. These low thyroid hormone levels have been documented using the PBI, serum thyroxine and serum total T_3 levels.

During acute infections it can be shown that there are striking changes in thyroid function with a fall in both the serum total T_4 and T_3 values with increasing levels of free thyroid hormones (Lutz et al., 1972). These changes have therefore been attributed to changes in the binding capacity, particularly TBPA.

These studies in acute infection are in keeping with studies by Jeffereys et al. (1972) in a prospective study of geriatric patients admitted to an acute geriatric hospital. It was found there that the low PBI correlated with severity of illness rather than age of the patient and the changes in PBI paralleled changes in serum albumin, suggesting that this was a protein binding effect. However, in our studies of healthy old people at home there was no correlation between the PBI and serum albumin. Most recent studies have shown a consistent pattern of thyroid hormone changes in acute illness. This is that the serum thyroxine value is usually slightly low, while the serum T_3 value is strikingly low and indeed may approach undetectable levels. At the same time the reverse T_3 value is elevated (Burrows et al., 1977). This seems to be a protective mechanism to help to guard against any undue metabolic effects of high free hormone levels during an acute illness.

This pattern of tests has been found not only in illness but also in malnutrition. It has been found in kwashiorkor and in anorexia nervosa, although in some personal studies in milder degrees of dietary amenorrhoea low serum T_3 values were found without any compensatory increase in free T_3 (Thomson et al., 1977). Similar effects can be shown during therapeutic starvation in the management of gross obesity (Vagenakis, 1977) and in this type of study it is interesting that the critical factor appears to be the amount of carbohydrate in the diet. The converse finding of elevated serum T_3 levels with rapid weight gain has also been shown (Bray et al., 1976).

Another organ of obvious importance in thyroid hormone control is the liver, because the liver is not only the site of manufacture of TBG and TBPA but also it is an important site of thyroxine metabolism. Indeed studies have suggested that as much as 30 per cent of the thyroxine in the body outside the thyroid gland is in the liver and that this acts as a pool of exchangeable thyroxine. Thyroxine is metabolized in the liver by conjugation and excretion into the biliary tract. On the other hand T_3 is not usually conjugated but tends to be sulphated and mainly excreted by the kidney. In keeping with the differences are studies by McConnon et al. (1972), which showed that in patients with cirrhosis there was a normal total T_4 and T_3 level with an elevated serum free T_4 and T_3 level. The production rate for T_4 was diminished but for T_3 was elevated. TBG capacity was increased but TBPA diminished. This study, therefore, seemed to confirm that the liver was very important in thyroxine metabolism, but less so in T_3 metabolism.

Likewise in renal disease abnormalities of thyroid hormone metabolism have been reported. Some of these can be easily explained such as the low TBG values with subsequent low serum T_4 and T_3 levels found in patients with the nephrotic syndrome due to excretion of TBG in the urine. In other patients with renal disease, however, a variety of changes in the thyroid function tests can be found (Gomez-Pan et al., 1979); but usually the use of corrected thyroxine value will ensure a result consistent with the clinical status (Joasoo et al., 1974).

Influence of Drugs

Many drugs have been shown to alter thyroid function tests in various ways. Leaving aside the therapeutic antithyroid drugs such as carbimazole and thiouracil, very few drugs exert a clinically significant effect on intrathyroidal hormone metabolism. Perhaps the two which are most significant are lithium and iodine. Lithium alters hormone release from the thyroid and has been associated with clinical hypothyroidism and also paradoxically with clinical thyrotoxicosis (Brownlie et al., 1976).

In certain susceptible patients large doses of iodide have a thiouracil-like effect and can result in goitrous hypothyroidism. This is seen particularly in the fetal thyroid where the mother is taking therapeutic doses of iodides; but it can also be seen in the adult. Indeed in one study (Jubiz et al., 1977) of 13 patients with chronic obstructive airways disease on iodides all had a low level of serum T_4 with an elevated TSH. This was not seen in experimental studies in normal individuals, which may reflect differences in the duration of treatment. There has been recent interest in the effect of iodides in radiological preparations on thyroid function. These have been recognized to be able to precipitate thyrotoxicosis in predisposed individuals, but one drug in particular (sodium iopanoate) has been recognized to increase the serum T_4, reverse T_3 and TSH concentrations and diminish the serum T_3 without causing clinical thyroid dysfunction (Burgi et al., 1976).

In addition to the above drugs, many drugs such as thiocyanate, sulphonylureas and sulphonamides can be shown experimentally to have minor effects on the thyroid. There is usually no clinical disease resulting from their administration.

Many drugs have the effect of altering the peripheral metabolism of the thyroid hormones. The drugs affecting the protein bound iodine have been reviewed by Davis (1966). Many of the drugs affecting this test did so due to associated iodine contamination, but in addition the PBI estimation reflects the level of the serum thyroxine and it was recognized that drugs such as oestrogens regularly increased the serum thyroxine by increasing TBG levels and that conversely the androgens and antiepileptic drugs, in particular phenytoin, lowered the serum thyroxine value. It was originally considered that this latter effect was simply due to alteration of protein binding because it could be shown *in vitro*, particularly, with phenytoin. However, subsequent studies have also shown that phenytoin alters the degradation of thyroxine by enzyme induction in the liver, and this is thought to be the main way in which the serum thyroxine is lowered when the drug is used therapeutically. The same effect has been found with phenobarbitone, a drug which has been in use for many years in the management of thyrotoxicosis and was thought purely to have a sedative action.

Recently it has been recognized that drugs may not only alter the degradation of the thyroid hormones but may affect their metabolism in the plasma or peripheral tissues. Propylthiouracil (PTU) appears to inhibit the peripheral conversion of thyroxine to triiodothyronine (Oppenheimer et al., 1972) and this might be of value in the control of clinical thyrotoxicosis. Recent work has shown that propranolol which was thought to act purely as an antiadrenergic agent and thus control the peripheral manifestations of thyrotoxicosis also seems to alter the metabolism of thyroxine, giving decreased levels of serum T_3 and increased levels of reverse T_3 (Harrower et al., 1977).

Another possible mechanism of altering the peripheral metabolism of thyroid hormones is by means of effects on hepatic binding. It will be remembered that the liver contains a significant store of thyroxine which is capable of interchanging with the plasma thyroxine. It has been recognized that heparin elevates the total thyroxine and free thyroxine values when administered *in vivo* either to normal subjects or even to patients who are on thyroxine therapy. This is not an assay problem since it does not interfere *in vitro* with the assay procedure. The demonstration of the same effect in athyreotic subjects on replacement therapy indicates that the thyroid gland itself is not involved in this process, and is supportive evidence for the thyroxine coming from some other pool, of which the liver is much the most likely (Saeed-Uz-Zafar et al., 1971).

Some drugs have a very complex effect on the hypothalamic-pituitary-thyroid system. As an example of this, large doses of steroids diminish TSH and its response to TRH and also decrease total and free serum T_3 without affecting T_4 values (Re et al., 1976).

Cholestyramine has a very interesting effect. Because of increasing binding of the thyroid hormones in the gastrointestinal tract it causes increased faecal loss of thyroxine and therefore increased requirement of thyroid hormone. This effect has been recognized as being of significance in patients who are requiring both therapeutic cholestyramine and thyroxine, in whom it has been recommended that either a larger dose of thyroxine should be given or, alternatively, there should be a delay between the administration of the two drugs.

REFERENCES

Bray G. A., Fisher D. A. and Chopra I. J. (1976) *Lancet* 1, 1206.
Brownlie B. E. W., Chambers S. T., Sadler W. A. et al. (1976) *Aust. NZ J. Med.* 6, 223.
Burgi H., Wimpfheimer C., Burger A. et al. (1976) *J. Clin. Endocrinol. Metab.* 43, 1203.
Burrows A. W., Cooper E., Shakespear R. A. et al. (1977) *Clin. Endocrinol.* 7, 289.

Burrows A. W., Shakespear R. A., Hesch R. D. et al. (1975) *Br. Med. J.* **4**, 437.
Davis P. J. (1966) *Am. J. Med.* **40**, 918.
Evered D. C., Tunbridge W. M. G., Hall R. et al. (1978) *Clin. Chim. Acta* **83**, 223.
Gaffney G. W., Gregerman R. I. and Shock N. W. (1962) *J. Clin. Endocrinol. Metab.* **22**, 784.
Gomez-Pan A., Alvarez-Ude F. et al. (1979) *Clin. Endocrinol.* **11**, 567.
De Groot L. J. and Niepomniszcze H. (1977) *Metabolism* **26**, 665.
Hansen J. M., Skovsted L. and Siersboek-Nielsen K. (1975) *Acta Endocrinol.* **79**, 60.
Harrower A. D. B., Fyffe J. A., Horn D. B. et al. (1977) *Clin. Endocrinol.* **7**, 41.
Herrmann J., Rusche H. J., Kroll H. J. et al. (1974) *Horm. Metab. Res.* **6**, 239.
Jeffereys P. M., Farran H. E. A., Hoffenberg R. et al. (1972) *Lancet* **1**, 924.
Joasoo A., Murray I. P. C., Parkin J. et al. (1974) *Q. J. Med.* **43**, 245.
Jubiz W., Carlile S. and Lagerquist L. D. (1977) *J. Clin. Endocrinol. Metab.* **44**, 379.
Lutz J. H., Gregerman R. I., Spaulding S. W. et al. (1972) *J. Clin. Endocrinol. Metab.* **35**, 230.
McConnon J., Row V. V. and Volpe R. (1972) *J. Clin. Endocrinol. Metab.* **34**, 144.
Ohara H., Kobayashi T., Shiraishi M. et al. (1974) *Endocrinol. Jpn.* **21**, 377.
Olsen T., Laurberg P. and Weeke J. (1978) *J. Clin. Endocrinol. Metab.* **47**, 1111.
Oppenheimer J. H., Schwartz H. L. and Surks M. (1972) *J. Clin. Invest.* **51**, 2493.
Ratcliffe W. A., Marshall J. and Ratcliffe J. G. (1976) *Clin. Endocrinol.* **5**, 631.
Re R. N., Kourides I. A., Ridgway E. C. et al. (1976) *J. Clin. Endocrinol. Metab.* **43**, 338.
Robbins J. (1975) In: Jamieson G. A. and Greenwalt T. J. (ed.), *Progress in Clinical and Biological Research, Vol. 5.* New York, Liss, p. 331.
Saeed-Uz-Zafar M., Miller J. M., Breneman G. M. et al. (1971) *J. Clin. Endocrinol. Metab.* **32**, 633.
Snyder P. J. and Utiger R. D. (1972) *J. Clin. Endocrinol. Metab.* **34**, 380.
Stanbury J. B. and Talley D. (1977) *Pharmacol. Ther. C.* **2**, 167.
Thomson J. A., Andrews G. R., Caird F. I. et al. (1972) *Age Ageing* **1**, 158.
Thomson J. E., Baird S. G. and Thomson J. A. (1977) *Clin. Endocrinol.* **7**, 383.
Tucker R. G. and Keys A. (1951) *J. Clin. Invest.* **30**, 869.
Vagenakis A. G. (1977) In: Virersky R. A. (ed.), *Anorexia Nervosa.* New York, Raven, p. 243.

17. THYROID DISORDERS
M. Hodkinson

HYPOTHYROIDISM

Hypothyroidism is a common condition in old age. Indeed, after diabetes mellitus, it is the commonest endocrine disorder in the age group. Unfortunately, not all patients present with classic signs and symptoms so that the routine use of laboratory screening tests, such as serum T_4 (thyroxine) and T_3 (triiodothyronine) uptake, or else a very high degree of clinical suspicion, are needed if many cases are not to be missed and so denied the benefits of treatment.

Aetiology and Prevalence

Most cases of hypothyroidism in old age are thought to be of autoimmune origin, cases due to hypopituitarism being very rarely encountered in the elderly. However iatrogenic causes are quite important, since hypothyroidism quite often follows surgical or radioiodine treatment for previous thyrotoxicosis. Antithyroid drugs may also be responsible. This effect is unlikely to be overlooked when such drugs have been given in thyrotoxicosis, but the antithyroid effects of lithium carbonate given in manic-depressive psychosis need to be remembered.

Relapse of hypothyroidism due to discontinuation of treatment is also often seen in the elderly. The patient may become forgetful and unreliable, or the drug is discontinued by the doctor who perhaps disbelieves the diagnosis made many years before, or overlooks the need to continue maintenance therapy when more recent medical events and their treatment occupy his attention.

Hypothyroidism in elderly patients is associated with other autoimmune conditions. Thus the prevalence of hypothyroidism in female geriatric patients without other autoimmune disease is estimated to be 1·7 per cent, but is 6 per cent in those with pernicious anaemia and 7 per cent in those with rheumatoid arthritis (Hodkinson, 1977). There is a similar picture in elderly men, though prevalences are all considerably lower (0·6 per cent cf. 1·2 and 1·6 per cent). Thyroid disease (hypo- and hyperthyroidism) is also associated with Addison's disease and vitiligo (Bahemuka and Hodkinson, 1975) and cranial arteritis (Thomas and Croft, 1974).

Clinical Presentation

The application of routine laboratory screening tests of thyroid function to series of elderly hospital patients (Jefferys, 1972; Bahemuka and

211

Hodkinson, 1975) gives a view of the clinical presentation of hypothyroidism which is not biased by preconceptions derived from the classic descriptions. These studies indicate that classic presentations occur in only a minority of elderly patients with hypothyroidism. Bahemuka and Hodkinson (1975) found that only a quarter of their series of elderly hypothyroid patients diagnosed by routine screening were clinically suspected on the basis of 'typical' signs and symptoms such as cold intolerance, hair loss, voice change, skin coarsening, or characteristic facies. Three-quarters had atypical clinical pictures. Of these, a quarter had wholly non-specific presentations with an insidious decline in general health and mobility, a half had a non-specific picture coupled with an associated autoimmune disease or a specific symptom such as reversible deafness, arthralgia or carpal tunnel syndrome, and the final quarter had psychiatric manifestations. Depression was by far the most common of these, paranoid states and delirium being less usual. Reversible dementia due to hypothyroidism (Granville-Grossman, 1971) did not occur in the series, nor was there any excess of non-reversible dementia when the series was compared with age- and sex-matched euthyroid admissions. Other relatively uncommon but important presentations of hypothyroidism in old age include coma associated with generalized convulsions and sometimes severe headache (Impallomeni, 1977), and hypothermia.

Physical Signs

The characteristic facies of myxoedema which can be so useful in the diagnosis of hypothyroidism in younger patients is of far less value in the elderly, since it can so readily be confused with the facial appearances of old age itself. Hair loss similarly is of little value. The most useful signs in old age are thus the voice change, a deep and croaky voice which can be quite characteristic, and the delay of the relaxation phase of tendon reflexes – the 'hung-up' reflex. The 'hung-up' reflex is not specific since it occurs in hypothermia, where it is thus of no value as an indication of possible hypothyroidism. Similarly bradycardia is common in hypothyroidism, but is a late and rather uncommon feature in old age.

Clinical goitre is an infrequent accompaniment of hypothyroidism in elderly patients, though at post-mortem a proportion will be found to have small multinodular goitres rather than thyroid atrophy (Bahemuka and Hodkinson, 1975). Effusions into body cavities are a rare manifestation of hypothyroidism (Sachdev and Hall, 1975), except that reversible deafness may be due to effusion into the middle ear in some cases.

Ischaemic heart disease is often associated with hypothyroidism. Indeed, premyxoedema appears to be a risk factor for the development of ischaemic heart disease (Fowler, 1977).

Treatment of Hypothyroidism

The treatment of hypothyroidism is with L-thyroxine. The use of the more rapidly acting triiodothyronine (T_3) or of T_4/T_3 mixtures confers no advantages and probably leads to a greater risk of iatrogenic thyrotoxicosis if doses are not carefully controlled. Thyroid extract is definitely contra-indicated because of its biological variability.

It is very important to start replacement therapy cautiously in the elderly patient as there is a risk of precipitating a myocardial infarction where ischaemic heart disease coexists. It is usual to begin with a daily dose of 0·05 mg and to increase this at intervals of a fortnight or longer until a satisfactory maintenance dose is reached. Adequacy of the dose can be assessed clinically or, more reliably, by laboratory tests. The most useful test is serum thyrotrophin (TSH) which falls to normal once the hypo-thyroidism is receiving adequate treatment. Evered and his colleagues (1973) have shown that few adults with hypothyroidism require more than 0·15 mg L-thyroxine per day to suppress TSH; the larger doses conventionally given in the past often lead to subclinical hyperthyroidism. Certainly most elderly patients require only 0·1 or 0·15 mg L-thyroxine per day.

Measurement of serum T_4 and T_3-uptake and calculation of the free thyroxine index (FTI) can also be used to monitor therapy. It is usual to adjust the dose of L-thyroxine so as to maintain a FTI in the upper part of the normal range.

Relapse of hypothyroidism due to lapse of treatment is seen with regrettable frequency in elderly patients. This emphasizes the need for supervision by the responsible doctor to ensure that treatment is main-tained for the remainder of the patient's life. Where patient compliance is poor because of depression or confusion, supervision by a neighbour, relative, or health visitor is necessary. The appropriateness of the mainten-ance dose of L-thyroxine should be checked from time to time by laboratory tests.

THYROTOXICOSIS

Thyrotoxicosis is less common than hypothyroidism in old age but is even more likely to present atypically. Indeed, the classic presentation with heat intolerance, hyperdynamic circulation, hot sweaty hands, tremor, diffuse goitre and eye signs is rarely seen. Diagnostic indices based on symptoms and signs such as Wayne's Index (Gurney et al., 1970), though of consider-able value in younger age groups, are virtually valueless in old age. The need for a high index of suspicion or the utilization of routine laboratory screening tests, already mentioned in the context of hypothyroidism, is even greater in the case of thyrotoxicosis in the elderly, particularly as failure to make the diagnosis can have more serious consequences for the patient.

Aetiology and Prevalence

The aetiology of thyrotoxicosis in the elderly is much the same as in younger age groups. Graves' disease with diffuse thyroid enlargement, and toxic multinodular goitre, account for the great majority of cases, thyrotoxicosis due to an autonomous toxic adenoma being far less common. In many patients the goitre may be clinically inapparent. The complex autoimmune mechanisms involved in the development of thyrotoxicosis are well reviewed by Hoffenberg (1974) and Kendall-Taylor (1975). The association of thyroid disease with other autoimmune diseases has already been detailed.

Bahemuka and Hodkinson (1975) applied routine laboratory screening tests to 2000 elderly patients admitted to a geriatric department and found 1·1 per cent of patients to have thyrotoxicosis. This is significantly higher than the 0·5 per cent found by Lloyd and Goldberg (1961) in a series of over 3000 geriatric admissions studied before screening tests were routinely available, and thus serves to underline the difficulties of clinical recognition of thyrotoxicosis in old age. This is further borne out by the findings of Rønnov-Jessen and Kirkegaard (1973), who showed that the proportion of all adults diagnosed as having thyrotoxicosis by a district service who were over the age of 60 rose substantially when the criteria for instituting thyroid investigations were broadened. The additional cases of thyrotoxicosis were mostly atypical in type. Their work also shows that thyrotoxicosis is considerably more common in the elderly than in the young. There is a female preponderance in old age as in younger age groups.

Forms of thyrotoxicosis in which serum T_3 is raised whilst serum T_4 remains within the normal range are now well recognized and have been designated T_3-toxicosis. This form of the disease has been reported in the elderly (Jefferys, 1972). However there seems no sound basis for this distinction from other cases of thyrotoxicosis in which both T_3 and T_4 are raised. Indeed, T_3-toxicosis may merely be an earlier stage in the development of the disease and is accompanied by no differences in aetiology, symptoms or signs (Editorial, *Br. Med. J.* 1972).

Clinical Presentation

The infrequent occurrence of the classic presentation of thyrotoxicosis in old age has been noted above. Rønnov-Jessen and Kirkegaard (1973) found the presentation to be classic in 47 per cent of patients aged 60—69 and in only 36 per cent of patients over 70. In their remaining patients, weight loss, anorexia, gastrointestinal symptoms, malaise and cardiovascular symptoms predominated. Hodkinson (1975), in a series of 22 patients with an average age of 80 who were diagnosed as thyrotoxic by routine screening, found that only 14 per cent presented classically. The remaining 86 per cent could be regarded as examples of 'masked thyrotoxicosis' (Editorial, *Lancet,* 1970). The commonest presentations were cardiovascular (heart failure 23 per cent, atrial fibrillation 9 per cent, sinus tachycardia 9 per cent). There was an association with pernicious anaemia in 9 per cent, and a clinical goitre in 4 per cent. However 32 per cent of cases had only the most general of symptoms such as weight loss and malaise.

Many authors agree that thyroid eye signs and goitre are far less common in the elderly thyrotoxic. Indeed, ophthalmoplegia, severe exophthalmos, pretibial myxoedema and thyroid acropachy are all considerable rarities in old age. Lid retraction is fairly common in elderly patients with thyrotoxicosis, but very similar appearances are far more often seen in euthyroid elderly patients with Parkinson's disease or pseudobulbar palsy.

Apathetic thyrotoxicosis (Lahey, 1931) is a clinical variant of thyrotoxicosis which is recognized as being particularly common in old age (Editorial, *Lancet*, 1970). Mental changes of slowness, apathy or depression tend to be prominent. Typical eye signs are usually absent but ptosis may occur. Severe weight loss and weakness are common and the proximal myopathy which may accompany any type of thyrotoxicosis, is often particularly severe. Atrial fibrillation is often present and many cases go on to develop cardiac failure. Patients may lapse into stupor or coma or alternatively may develop thyroid crisis.

Untreated thyrotoxicosis in old age is a serious threat to life. Recognition of the atypical case is thus of considerable importance. Death from cardiac failure is particularly important, tachycardia being an adverse prognostic sign. Other causes of death are thyroid crisis and coma in the apathetic case. Thromboembolic deaths are also quite frequent, and a number of patients die from no obvious cause other than their hypermetabolic state (Parker and Lawson, 1973).

Treatment of Thyrotoxicosis

The choice of treatment for the elderly thyrotoxic patient lies between antithyroid drugs, radioactive iodine and thyroidectomy. Surgical treatment by partial thyroidectomy is seldom used in old age unless there is a goitre which is giving rise to pressure symptoms. The choice thus usually lies between antithyroid drugs and radioactive iodine, and the advantages and disadvantages are fairly evenly balanced.

Antithyroid Drugs

In Britain carbimazole is most often used, starting with a dose of 40—60 mg/d. Carbimazole is a short acting drug and so needs to be given 6—8-hourly; good patient compliance is thus essential. Thyroid function is monitored frequently by serum T_4 and T_3 uptake tests. As soon as the FTI falls to the normal range, the dose of carbimazole is reduced to the smallest dose which will control the FTI. This maintenance dose is usually 2·5—5 mg 8-hourly. Euthyroid status is usually achieved within a few weeks of commencing treatment. Regular follow-up is required to regulate the maintenance dose and to look out for the infrequent occurrence of sensitivity rashes or the very rare complication of agranulocytosis; both usually occur in the first month of treatment.

Patients with toxic multinodular goitre usually require permanent therapy but those with Graves' disease have an approximately 50 per cent chance of being in remission if carbimazole is stopped after 1–2 years. However subsequent relapse may occur even after many years off treatment so that long term follow-up will still be required.

Of the other antithyroid drugs, methylthiouracil and propylthiouracil are very similar therapeutically and in terms of the incidence of side effects, and may replace carbimazole in patients who develop side effects. Potassium perchlorate is best avoided as there is a much greater risk of agranulocytosis.

Radioactive Iodine

Radioactive iodine therapy uses ^{131}I, ^{125}I having been found to have no advantages. It is an inexpensive treatment which calls for minimum patient cooperation in that it is simply administered as a single oral dose in aqueous solution. Furthermore, earlier fears of possible carcinogenic or leukaemogenic effects have not been substantiated despite its large scale use. Against this, however, it is far slower in its action and takes 2–3 months to render the patient euthyroid. It is also very difficult to find the right dose. If too little is given, repeat doses will be necessary, and the patient may be inadequately treated for many months. Too large a dose will lead to hypothyroidism and the need for permanent thyroxine replacement therapy. Even where initial dosage is satisfactory there is a steady risk of the later development of hypothyroidism at a rate of approximately 5 per cent per year.

Radioactive iodine should not be given where a goitre is retrosternal or is giving rise to tracheal displacement, as there may be some temporary enlargement of the gland within the first ten days of treatment.

Radioactive iodine therapy is thus more suited to the milder case of thyrotoxicosis. As with carbimazole therapy, permanent follow-up is indicated because of the risk of subsequent development of hypothyroidism. There is however virtually no risk of recurrence of thyrotoxicosis once the patient has been made euthyroid.

Nodular Goitre in Old Age

Clinically apparent goitre is quite uncommon in elderly patients in iodine-sufficient areas. Nonetheless, post-mortem studies in such non-goitre areas show that small nodular goitres are common. Denham and Wills (1980) finding 27 per cent in a geriatric series in London. Much higher figures of 50 per cent or more are reported from iodine-deficient areas.

The high prevalence of nodular glands is likely to be of some importance. It may well underlie the greatly increased vulnerability of the elderly to the development of iodine-induced thyrotoxicosis, which is discussed below. Denham and Wills (1980) also found that nodularity was associated with a higher frequency of borderline elevations and reductions of FTI in life. This suggests that there may be an important link between nodularity of the thyroid gland and the high incidence of both hypothyroidism and thyrotoxicosis in old people.

Iodine-induced Thyrotoxicosis

Iodine-induced thyrotoxicosis (the Jod—Basedow phenomenon) has been recognized for more than 150 years. Thyrotoxicosis develops when iodides are administered to patients with goitre in endemic goitre areas (Hoffenberg, 1974). Similarly, small amounts of iodine such as those introduced into the diet by the iodisation of salt have given rise to epidemics of thyrotoxicosis in goitrous areas such as Tasmania (Stewart and Vidor, 1976). These authors found that there was a rising vulnerability to iodine-induced thyrotoxicosis at higher ages.

However, iodine may also induce thyrotoxicosis in goitre patients in non-goitre areas. This occurred in four of eight Boston goitre patients given large doses of iodide (Vagenakis et al., 1972). Denham and Himsworth (1974) showed that this can very readily occur when iodides are given in moderate amounts to elderly patients without clinically apparent goitre or previous thyroid disease. Potassium iodide given to block the thyroid during ^{125}I-fibrinogen screening for venous thrombosis in 29 previously euthyroid geriatric patients resulted in three of them becoming thyrotoxic; they had encountered three other cases before this prospective study. One patient came to post mortem and was found to have a nodular thyroid gland. As there was a 27 per cent prevalence of nodular thyroid in a geriatric post-mortem series from the same hospital (Denham and Wills, 1978), it seems likely that the remaining cases also had clinically inapparent nodular goitres.

Iodine-induced thyrotoxicosis is probably very common in elderly patients who may receive substantial amounts of iodine either as drugs or in the form of radiological contrast media, e.g. during cholecystography or intravenous pyelography. Fortunately iodine-induced thyrotoxicosis is usually fairly mild and self-limiting, thyroid function typically returning to normal within three months once iodine is discontinued. However this is not always so, and some cases may have quite marked symptoms and require antithyroid drugs for a time (Denham and Himsworth, 1974).

REFERENCES

Bahemuka M. and Hodkinson H. M. (1975) *Br. Med. J.* 2, 601.
Denham M. J. and Himsworth R. L. (1974) *Age Ageing* 3, 221.
Denham M. J. and Wills E. J. (1980) *Gerontology* 26, 160.
Editorial (1972) *Br. Med. J.* 2, 306.
Editorial (1970) *Lancet* 2, 809.
Evered D., Young E. T., Ormston B. J. et al. (1973) *Br. Med. J.* 3, 131.
Fowler P. B. S. (1977) *Proc. R. Soc. Med.* 70, 297.
Granville-Grossman K. (1971) *Recent Advances in Clinical Psychiatry.* London, Churchill, p. 219.
Gurney C., Owen S. G., Hall R. A. et al. (1970) *Lancet* 2, 1275.
Hodkinson H. M. (1975) *Diagnostic and Prognostic Aspects of Routine Laboratory Screening in the Geriatric In-patient.* D M Thesis, University of Oxford.

Hodkinson H. M. (1977) *Biochemical Diagnosis of the Elderly*. London, Chapman & Hall, p. 76.
Hoffenberg R. (1974) *Br. Med. J.* **3**, 452.
Impallomeni M. G. (1977) *Age Ageing* **6**, 71.
Jefferys P. M. (1972) *Age Ageing* **1**, 33.
Kendall-Taylor P. (1975) *Br. J. Hosp. Med.* **12**, 638.
Lahey F. H. (1931) *New Eng. J. Med.* **204**, 747.
Lloyd W. H. and Goldberg I. J. L. (1961) *Br. Med. J.* **1**, 1208.
Parker J. L. W. and Lawson D. H. (1973) *Lancet* **2**, 894.
Rønnov-Jessen V. and Kirkegaard C. (1973) *Br. Med. J.* **1**, 41.
Sachdev Y. and Hall R. (1975) *Lancet* **1**, 564.
Stewart J. C. and Vidor G. I. (1976) *Br. Med. J.* **1**, 372.
Thomas R. D. and Croft D. N. (1974) *Br. Med. J.* **2**, 408.
Vagenakis A. G., Braverman L. E., Ingbar S. H. et al. (1972) *Lancet* **2**, 1421.

GENERAL REFERENCES

DHSS (1969) *Recommended Intakes of Nutrients for the United Kingdom. Report on Public Health and Medical Subjects* No. 120. London, HMSO.

DHSS (1970) *First Report by the Panel on Nutrition of the Elderly. Report on Public Health and Medical Subjects* No. 123. London, HMSO.

DHSS (1972) *A Nutrition Survey of the Elderly. Report on Public Health and Medical Subjects* No. 3. London, HMSO.

Exton-Smith A. N. and Scott D. L. (ed.) (1968) *Vitamins in the Elderly.* Bristol, Wright.

Fielding J. (ed.) (1976) *Ferastral: Iron-poly (sorbitol gluconic acid) complex: Proceedings of a Conference, London, Scand. J. Haematol.* Suppl. 32.

KEHF (1965) Exton-Smith A. N. and Stanton B. R. *Report of an Investigation into the Dietary of Elderly Women Living Alone.* London, King Edward's Hospital Fund.

KEHF (1972) Exton-Smith A. N., Stanton B. R. and Windsor A. C. M. (1972) *Nutrition of Housebound Old People.* London, King Edward's Hospital Fund.

Kief H. (ed.) *Iron Metabolism and its Disorders.* Amsterdam, Excerpta Medica.

NAS/NRC (1964; 1974; 1978; 1979; 1980) National Research Council, Food and Nutrition Board *Recommended Dietary Allowances.* Washington DC, National Academy of Sciences.

Pories W. J., Strain W. H., Hsu J. M. et al. (ed.), *Clinical Applications of Zinc Metabolism.* Springfield, Thomas.

Prasad A. S. (1977) *Trace Elements in Human Health and Disease* Vol. 1. New York, Academic.

WHO/FAO (1973) *Energy and Protein Requirements. Report of a Joint FAO/WHO Ad Hoc Expert Committee. World Health Organization Report Series* No. 522. Geneva, WHO.

Index